60
WAYS
TO LOSE
10 Pounds
(or More)

ROBERT D. LESSLIE, MD

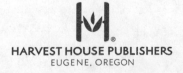

HARVEST HOUSE PUBLISHERS
EUGENE, OREGON

Cover by Koechel Peterson & Associates, Minneapolis, Minnesota

Some material in this book was previously published in Dr. Lesslie's book *60 Ways to Lower Your Cholesterol*.

This book is not intended to take the place of sound professional medical advice. Neither the author nor the publisher assumes any liability for possible adverse consequences as a result of the information contained herein.

Unless otherwise noted, the stories in this book are fictitious accounts used for illustration purposes only. Although based on the author's experiences, they are not meant to refer to any person, living or dead.

60 WAYS TO LOSE 10 POUNDS (OR MORE)
Copyright © 2016 Robert D. Lesslie, MD
Published by Harvest House Publishers
Eugene, Oregon 97402
www.harvesthousepublishers.com

ISBN 978-0-7369-6693-1 (pbk.)
ISBN 978-0-7369-6694-8 (eBook)

Library of Congress Cataloging-in-Publication Data
  Names: Lesslie, Robert D., 1951- author.
  Title: 60 ways to lose 10 pounds (or more) / Robert D. Lesslie, MD.
  Other titles: Sixty ways to lose ten pounds or more
  Description: Eugene, Oregon : Harvest House Publishers, [2016]
  Identifiers: LCCN 2016006023 | ISBN 9780736966931 (pbk.)
  Subjects: LCSH: Weight loss—Popular works.
  Classification: LCC RM222.2 .L4266 2016 | DDC 613.2/5—dc23 LC record available at
  http://lccn.loc.gov/2016006023

Printed in the United States of America

16 17 18 19 20 21 22 23 24 / BP-GL / 10 9 8 7 6 5 4 3 2 1

This book is dedicated to the many patients and friends who have encouraged me by their example and determination to lose weight and improve their health.

We can get there.

Contents

1. Dave Jernigan.   7

2. What's the Big Deal?.   10

3. Obesity and Heart Disease   13

4. Obesity and the Development of Diabetes   16

5. Obesity and Some Other Bad Stuff   19

6. The Metabolic Syndrome: When It All Goes Wrong   22

7. A Brief History of Weight Loss.   26

8. Setting a Goal.   30

9. Getting It Right: Jakey Taylor.   32

10. Let's Get Started!   35

11. Keeping a Food Journal   40

12. What's This Waist-Hip Ratio Business?:
    Comparing Apples to Pears   44

13. The Lowly Calorie: Unloved, Unappreciated,
    Yet So Important   47

14. Exercise, Part 1: Ya Gotta Get Movin'   51

15. Exercise, Part 2: Overcoming the Yo-Yo   54

16. Getting It Wrong: Sarah Hoffman   58

17. Discipline: A Muscle in Need of Exercise   62

18. Water, Water Everywhere...   64

19. What Am I Supposed to Be Eating?   68

20. What Diet Choices Are There?   70

21. The Fad Diets: They Come and Go   73

22. Why Low-Fat Diets Don't Work 77

23. The Low-Carbohydrate Approach 81

24. The Low-Carb Diet: What It Looks Like 85

25. What's the Best Diet?: One Clear Choice 88

26. The Mediterranean Diet: What It Looks Like. 91

27. "He Created Them Male and Female" 93

28. Getting It Wrong: Cindy Stewart 95

29. Complementary and Alternative Medicine (CAM) 100

30. CAM and Weight Loss: Dietary Supplements and
    What to Do with Them 103

31. Okay, Doc, I Think It's Time for a Pill 106

32. Prescription Weight-Loss Medicines:
    Is One Right for Me? 108

33. Prescription Weight-Loss Medicines, Part 1:
    Drugs That Alter Fat Digestion 111

34. Prescription Weight-Loss Medicines, Part 2:
    Serotonin Activators. 114

35. Prescription Weight-Loss Medicines, Part 3:
    The Stimulants 117

36. Prescription Weight-Loss Medicines, Part 4:
    The Combinations 120

37. The HCG Diet: Are We Really Still
    Talking About This? 123

38. Getting It Right: Isaac Dawkins 126

39. Commercial Weight-Loss Plans:
    Do They Work and Are They Worth It? 129

40. Jenny Craig 131

41. Weight Watchers 133

42. Nutrisystem 135

43. Bariatric Surgery, Part 1: What Are We Talking About?.... 137

44. Bariatric Surgery, Part 2: What Are Our Choices?........ 141

45. Bariatric Surgery, Part 3: The Pros, the Cons, and
    What You Can Expect 146

46. Choosing a Bariatric Surgeon:
    Does It Make a Difference? 151

47. Getting It Right: The Tortoise and the Hare............ 154

48. Eating Disorders, Part 1: Things You Need to Know...... 158

49. Eating Disorders, Part 2: Binge Eating 162

50. Eating Disorders, Part 3: Bulimia Nervosa 166

51. Eating Disorders, Part 4: Anorexia Nervosa 169

52. Getting It Wrong: George Winters 174

53. A Little Weight-Loss Potpourri..................... 178

54. Doctor, It's Just Got to Be Glandular 181

55. Frequently Asked Questions........................ 183

56. When You Reach the Plateau 188

57. Ghrelin and Leptin: The Future of Weight Loss? 192

58. A Little Perspective.............................. 195

59. Putting It All Together 198

60. Dave Jernigan: Victory! 202

    Some Final Thoughts 203

1

Dave Jernigan

Dave Jernigan had struggled with his weight for most of his 46 years. He had never been technically obese—maybe carrying an extra 10 or 20 pounds—but he felt as if he was always on a diet. He'd lose a few pounds, gain them back, then start over again. Nothing worked and nothing lasted. This time he was motivated—he had a reason to shed a few pounds.

"Dr. Lesslie, we've got my blood pressure under control now, with the medications you put me on a couple of months ago. And my cholesterol level is fine. But I'm not sure I want to keep taking those pills for the rest of my life. My wife and I have done the salt thing—really cutting back on adding any to our food and using the Lite Salt you recommended. I can do that forever. It's just the pills. What's the chance of being weaned off them?"

Dave had worked hard to get his lipids (his cholesterol level) under control and lower his blood pressure. And he had been successful, more so than many of our patients. He had done the most difficult part of all of this—taking a hard look at his lifestyle and making the appropriate changes. But if he wanted to limit the number of prescription medications he was taking, one more thing needed to happen.

I opened his chart and traced my finger over his vital signs, noted at the top of the page. His blood pressure was great—122/76. And his heart rate was where it needed to be—68. My finger came to rest over the box where the nurse had written his weight. I tapped it a couple of times and turned the record so Dave could see it.

"I know, I know, 212," he said. "I'm six feet one, and I guess I should weigh about…" He paused and patted his belly.

"A good target would be somewhere between 190 and 195," I told him.

"I was thinking more like 180," Dave said. "But I haven't seen that number since right after college."

I chuckled. "Well, we need to be realistic about a possible goal. Nothing worse than setting yourself up for failure. If you want to be aggressive, we can shoot for 190. That should be reachable."

"Speaking of realistic, Doc—if I can get down to that weight, what are the chances I'll be able to come off some of my blood pressure medicine? A friend of mine lost 30 pounds and his doctor stopped his BP meds *and* his cholesterol drug. That's where I'd like to be."

"That's impressive, Dave, especially if your friend has been able to keep that weight off. But back to your question about being realistic. If you can lose some weight—the 10 or 15 pounds we're talking about—there's a good chance we'll be able to adjust your medications. Nothing would make me happier, but it's not going to happen overnight. This is something you can do, but it will take some effort."

"I don't expect it to be easy, Doc, but how do we get started? What do I do now? I'm exercising about 45 minutes a day, four or five days a week, and pretty hard. Is that something I need to increase?"

"Not yet." I closed his chart and tossed it onto the countertop. "Let's start with something really simple, but you're going to have to be serious about it."

"What is it? I'm ready to get going today!"

"I want you to buy a notebook and starting keeping a diary of everything you eat."

His face dropped. "A diary? You've got to be kiddin' me, Doc. I want to get started with something exciting—some special diet or routine. Something challenging."

"Believe me, Dave—you do it right, you'll find keeping a food diary pretty challenging. But it's going to be critical if we're going to make this happen."

He shook his head and stared at the floor.

"Come back in two weeks with that diary," I told him. "Make sure you write down everything that goes into your mouth. Everything. Then we'll move on to something more exciting."

"Me, keeping a food diary," he muttered. "Who'd a thunk it?"

Okay, now it's time for me to get started too. I weighed this morning before eating or drinking anything and wrote down the number where I can find it. I hope. My plan is to increase my exercising by 10 or 15 minutes each day and cut down on my carbs. No more desserts on Sunday after church. And while I encouraged Dave to keep a food diary, I won't need to since I've been at this a while and know what I'm eating. Losing a pound a week is my goal. Shouldn't be too difficult.

2

What's the Big Deal?

For centuries, we've known that being overweight is bad for us. After all, it's one of the seven deadly sins, along with anger, envy, pride, and a few others. But just how bad is it? And why might this be important? We're going to consider the bad part, and I think it's important because if we really understand this, it will increase our motivation to do something about it. And that will prove to be key if we're going to be successful in losing weight and keeping it off.

Before we begin, we need to define some terms and keep them in mind. We'll find these throughout this book as reminders, just so we know what we're talking about.

First, we'll need to know our *body mass index* (BMI). We can easily find a calculator on the Internet to give us this number, but we'll first need to know our height and weight. (For a brief definition of BMI and a handy calculator to determine your BMI, go to: www.nhlbi.nih.gov/health/educational/lose_wt/BMI/bmicalc.htm.) Once we plug these numbers in, we'll have our BMI. Here are the standard definitions:

- The normal range is 18.5 to 25. (This is expressed as kilograms per meter squared. In this book, we're just going to use the numbers.)
- Overweight is a BMI of 25 to 29.9.
- Obesity is a BMI of 30 to 39.9.

- Severe obesity, or morbid obesity, is a BMI of greater than 40.

Now we know where we are, according to our BMI number and these definitions. But don't be discouraged. These are aggressive brackets, and you might find yourself overweight when you've been thinking you were just a few pounds heavier than you'd like to be. Most of us don't want to think of ourselves as being overweight—certainly not obese. But the number is right there in front of us. There is ongoing discussion about the accuracy and applicability of using our BMI for weight management, but at present, it's the best we have, and it's the standard by which our medical studies have been conducted.

Okay, now we've come to the "just how bad is it?" part. Here are the things we know:

- Being obese increases our risk of dying from any and all causes by more than 20 percent. (We will all one day die. We're talking about premature deaths.)
- Being severely obese increases the odds of dying even more—as much as 50-75 percent.
- Clear associations have been established for increased deaths due to various diseases when we are obese or severely obese. We're going to consider each of these in more detail, but the following are conditions with increased odds of dying when we're obese:
  - » Cardiovascular disease (heart attacks, stroke)
  - » Diabetes
  - » Cancers (this is especially true for those involving the breast, colon, prostate, liver, kidney, and uterus)
  - » Respiratory diseases (asthma and chronic obstructive pulmonary disease [COPD])

And if that's not enough to get our attention, here's what we know about life expectancy. When we're obese as adults (an age of 40 years or more), our expected lifespan will be reduced on average by 6 or 7 years compared to that of our friends who are of normal weight. Remember, that's at a BMI of greater than 30. If our number is somewhere between

25 and 29.9 (overweight), we can expect an average lifespan reduction of 3 years. Serious numbers and serious business. And just so you know how cigarette smoking impacts this, if you're obese and smoke, you're going to shorten your life by 13 or 14 years, when compared with nonsmokers who are normal weight.

One last sobering thought. We have enjoyed a gradual and steady rise in our life expectancies over the past couple of centuries. Some experts see that coming to a halt, largely due to the worldwide epidemic of obesity. We're not going to live forever, but if you're like me, I'd like to live as well as I can for as long as I can. That's why this is important.

Now we'll take a look at how being overweight impacts the diseases that afflict many of us and why this *is* such a big deal.

3

Obesity and Heart Disease

It might seem intuitive that being overweight would put us at risk for developing heart disease. But how might that happen? Let's start with what the experts have to say.

The American Heart Association (AHA) tells us that obesity is an *independent* risk factor for having various cardiovascular diseases. This means that in and of itself, being overweight puts us at risk. Obesity is certainly connected to other health concerns—high blood pressure, diabetes—which are also risk factors for heart disease. But being an independent risk factor should get our attention.

Okay, so what's the risk? How big a factor is this? In the ongoing Nurses' Health Study, more than 110,000 women have been followed for a couple of decades, and a multitude of health issues have been evaluated. One of these is the connection between a woman's BMI and her risk of dying from a cardiovascular disease (heart attack, heart failure, stroke). It turns out that among women with a BMI of 32 or higher, the risk of death is four times that of women with a BMI less than 19. Four times. That's a huge number.

Other studies have demonstrated a consistent association between obesity and the common cardiovascular diseases, but how does this happen? What's the underlying mechanism here? There appear to be several, all of which are related to changes in our metabolism and in the functioning of our organs, tissues, and cells that occurs as we gain weight and our

BMI creeps into the obese zone. Most of these make sense, while a few might be a little surprising.

First, obesity creates problems with the handling of our blood sugar and increasing complications with the hormone *insulin*. We'll talk more about that when we consider the association between obesity and diabetes, but for now, we need to know that being overweight frequently leads to insulin resistance and the overproduction of insulin. This simple chain of proteins can wreak havoc in several important areas of our bodies, including our heart and blood vessels.

When this insulin resistance reaches a critical point, our pancreas finally wears out and we develop full-blown diabetes. This disease itself is associated with the development of coronary artery disease and other serious vascular problems.

And then we have the lipid abnormalities that result from becoming obese. These include a low HDL level (the *good* cholesterol), increased levels of some of the harmful carriers of the cholesterol molecule, and increased levels of triglycerides (blood fats). All of these are known precipitants of heart and blood vessel disease.

Because of several physiologic changes in our bodies due to obesity, our blood pressure can rise. If we already have hypertension, this makes its management much more difficult. And as we know, high blood pressure is clearly associated with the development of cardiovascular disease. One of the physiologic changes seen with increasing weight is the development of "left ventricular hypertrophy." Simply stated, our heart muscle has to get larger in order to pump blood through a vascular bed that is getting bigger and bigger. This *hypertrophy* is not a good thing, and is a marker for heart attacks, heart failure, and sudden death.

We also know that obesity is linked to unhealthy blood vessels. The lining of our arteries—large and small—need to be smooth, glistening, and able to react to various stresses and internal signals by contracting and dilating when needed. This doesn't happen in those of us who are overweight, and this problem gets worse with time. It manifests itself in heart disease, but also in peripheral vascular diseases, which are circulation disorders that affect blood vessels outside the brain or heart, such as leg pain brought on by walking and other painful conditions.

For some reason, obesity is frequently related to abnormalities with the sympathetic nervous system. This is another of the physiologic changes that take place with increasing weight, and has to do with our "fight or flight" mechanism. Mainly this impacts the increased release of epinephrine (adrenaline) and can result in significant electrical problems within our hearts—principally development of arrhythmias, including atrial fibrillation. This is an all-too-frequent problem, and something we don't want if we can help it.

Then there's obstructive sleep apnea (OSA). Obesity is clearly related to the development of this problem, as demonstrated by the fact that weight loss is the single most important intervention in correcting this condition. If people with OSA are able to lose weight, they are frequently able to avoid surgery or CPAP machines. Once we have it though, OSA leads to an increase in mortality, high blood pressure, and cardiac arrhythmias (again, atrial fibrillation being one of the most common).

We mentioned the connection between obesity and heart failure (the inability of the heart muscle to pump enough blood to meet the body's needs). This is becoming an increasingly common problem, and you may know someone or have a family member with this disease. It's difficult to manage and something to avoid, if possible. There are many causes of congestive heart failure (CHF), but obesity is clearly one of them. Researchers tell us that the risk of CHF doubles when our BMI exceeds 30. It gets worse as we gain more weight. Specifically, for every BMI unit above 30, our risk for developing heart failure increases by about 5 percent. That's a lot, but thankfully it can be prevented.

As we can see, there's a clear and bothersome association between obesity and cardiovascular diseases. We probably knew that, but maybe not how bad it really is. If this is not motivating enough for us, we'll consider diabetes in the next chapter.

4

Obesity and the Development of Diabetes

In the previous chapter, we looked at the connection between obesity and heart disease. As with most of these associations, it's frequently difficult to differentiate the cart from the horse, or the chicken from the egg, or the... Well, you get the idea. Gaining excess weight doesn't happen in a vacuum, but stems from overeating, lack of exercise, genetics, poor life choices— many of the things that lead to heart disease, diabetes, and other degenerative and significant diseases we'll be considering.

So is it fair or even useful to point a finger at being overweight as a real health hazard? We showed that with heart disease, that is indeed the case. The same is true for diabetes. There is a clear association between obesity and the development of type 2 diabetes. But what is it, and how does it happen?

First, here's what we know. Type 2 diabetes (known as "adult onset diabetes") is strongly associated with obesity (remember, that's a BMI of greater than 30). This association reaches across all ethnic groups, and it's believed that at least 80 percent of all adult onset diabetes can be attributed to obesity. We need to stop and think about that for a moment. Eight out of every ten cases. That's a huge number and would indicate that something is going on here. Just what is that something?

It's become clear that obesity is linked with "impaired glucose tolerance"—the ability of our bodies to handle a carbohydrate load. This happens over time, and requires a near-constant intake of too much sugar and starch—the all-American diet. This intolerance of glucose is caused by several factors, and ultimately leads to the development of type 2 diabetes. One of these mechanisms has to do with the efficiency of insulin as it acts in our tissues to cause the uptake of glucose. This happens through the means of specialized receptors located on the walls of most of our cells. Over time, these receptors literally wear out from overuse, requiring more and more insulin to be released. This process occurs in the face of continued carbohydrate overloading, but the presence of obesity accelerates the decline in the functioning of these receptors. This appears to be "dose-related" in that the more we exceed our ideal weight, the more rapidly we develop insulin resistance. We're not exactly sure how this happens, but genetics seems to play a part. As does the distribution of our excess fat—whether it's around our waist or more generally located. We'll be talking about this issue later, and how it seems to affect several critical health factors.

Another way that obesity increases our chances of developing diabetes is through its known connection with increased mediators of inflammation. There are a bunch of these, and we won't list them all here. But you've heard and read about how inflammation can cause a whole host of problems. This is going to be one of those places, since we know that specific factors released from our fat cells stimulate inflammatory activity, leading to the development of type 2 diabetes (as well as atherosclerosis). As supportive proof for this theory, individuals taking strong anti-inflammatory drugs—such as those used in the treatment of psoriasis and rheumatoid arthritis—enjoy a markedly reduced risk of becoming diabetics. Again, obesity leads to the elevation of the agents of inflammation, which cause a bunch of bad things to happen in our bodies, which triggers the development of diabetes.

And lastly, we need to consider *leptin,* a naturally occurring chemical that helps us maintain a normal weight. You've probably read about this, and if not, you will in the near future. This is the cutting edge of weight loss, and we'll be taking a more in-depth look at it later on. For the present, we need to know that leptin is produced by our fat cells, and signals our brains when we've had enough to eat, thus causing us to exercise those muscles that push us away from the dinner table. That's the best-case scenario, when things are working properly. But in the presence of obesity, we can experience a deficiency in this chemical, or another of those "resistance" problems. Leptin is released and floating around in our body, but it doesn't pack the punch that it should, or once did. Again, cutting-edge stuff and pretty exciting. Just something to keep in mind as we consider the tools at our disposal in our struggle to lose weight.

And it is a struggle, but there's a lot of hope here. We know some of the linkage between obesity and the development of type 2 diabetes, and how one leads to the other. And we also know that as we lose weight and are no longer in the obese range, these factors—insulin resistance, inflammatory chemicals, leptin deficiency—all get better. That should be encouraging and add to our motivation.

5

Obesity and Some Other Bad Stuff

Okay, so we now know the connection between obesity and heart disease, as well as diabetes. That should be enough to get our attention and rev up our motivation to improve our health and lessen our odds of developing these two common and significant problems. But there are other things out there—other bad stuff—that are clearly linked to obesity. Let's consider the important ones.

Atrial fibrillation. While this might technically fall under the category of "heart disease," this problem deserves a little special attention. First, it's very common; second, it can cause devastating problems (strokes); and third, it may largely be preventable. We know that obese individuals have a 50 percent greater risk of developing this arrhythmia than those who fall in the normal or even overweight brackets. And we know that if we're obese and have atrial fibrillation, and we lose as little as 8 percent of our current weight, four out of five of us will see this rhythm problem improve and some will see it completely go away.

Gallbladder disease. If you've ever had gallstones or a gallbladder infection, you know this is serious business. A gallbladder attack changes everything, and quickly brings people to our office or to the ER. If you get the chance to take a pass on this problem, I'd recommend it. We know that the incidence of gallstones and gallbladder disease increases with increasing weight, with worsening obesity being associated with the greatest risk.

Stroke. This problem is more common in those of us who are obese, with a documented increased incidence of 10 to 20 percent. This is for the risk factor of obesity alone. When you factor in the things that are frequently associated with being overweight (elevated blood pressure, diabetes, elevated cholesterol), the odds really go up. No one wants a stroke, so we need to pay attention to this.

Arthritis. Obese individuals have a much higher incidence of osteoarthritis (the wearing away of our joints) than do those of us who are more lean. The most frequently affected areas are our knees and ankles—what you might expect with the added stress of excess weight pounding away at these joints. But we also see an increase in weight-related arthritis in other areas of our body, suggesting that something else is also at work here. The good news is that weight loss can be associated with a significant reduction in the risk of developing osteoarthritis and may even reverse some of the pain once it's established.

Various infections. The association between obesity and the increased risk of several infections has been clearly established. Largely these have to do with the skin, post-op infections, and respiratory infections (frequently pneumonia), especially during the flu season. While this connection is well established, we're not exactly sure of the mechanism. We mentioned the decreased levels of leptin in obesity, and this might be one of the players here. Increased inflammatory chemicals might play a part as well. Whatever the reason, obesity increases our susceptibility to many important infections. And once established, these infections are harder to clear in those of us who are overweight.

Respiratory problems. Several pulmonary issues are worsened or even caused by the presence of obesity. Obstructive sleep apnea is one of these and is a significant health hazard for many of us. We've mentioned the significance of this problem and the importance of having it accurately diagnosed and treated. Aggressive weight loss is the first line of treatment for sleep apnea, pointing out its causative potential. Another respiratory problem has to do with the simple mechanics of excess weight limiting our ability to fully inflate our lungs. This is a real concern in those of us with asthma, COPD, and other lung issues. Any reserve of lung function is lost, placing us at risk for low oxygen levels and increasing the risk of pneumonia, again simply due to the mechanical difficulty of ventilating our airways.

Cancer. Cancer and obesity? How could they possibly be connected? There are several theories as to how this happens, but for right now, we need to be aware that being obese carries with it an increased risk of developing certain cancers. The association is well established and includes the following types of malignancies:

uterine	prostate
breast	ovarian
colon	thyroid
gallbladder	some types of leukemia
liver	

How close is this linkage? It varies, depending on the type of cancer. For instance, it's believed that as much as 40 percent of uterine cancer is directly associated with a BMI greater than 35, while that number falls to about 2 to 3 percent with thyroid cancer. And with prostate cancer, obesity is associated with more aggressive tumors. The important point here is that obesity, for whatever reason, increases our risk for developing a wide range of cancers. Another motivational point.

And if that's not enough, we know that a high BMI is also associated with various kinds of kidney disease, kidney stones, irregular menses, and decreased fertility. And for you guys out there, obesity is an independent (meaning it does this on its own) risk factor for erectile dysfunction.

Plenty of reasons here to lose some weight. And while some of this information is relatively recent, the desire to trim and slim is nothing new. We've been trying to do this for centuries. We'll be taking a look at how our predecessors addressed this challenge, with varying degrees of success—and sometimes costly failure. But first, a close look at the dreaded metabolic syndrome.

6

The Metabolic Syndrome

When It All Goes Wrong

If you haven't heard of this, you probably will. In fact, you may have it. One in three of us does. *One in three.* That's a big number, especially when we consider the odds of dying from cancer (one in four), developing appendicitis (one in seven), or dying in an auto accident (one in seventy-five). And if the name doesn't sound serious enough, it wasn't very long ago that this was known as syndrome X. In fact, the Aussies aptly call this CHAOS (Coronary artery disease, Hypertension, Atherosclerosis, Obesity, and Stroke), and we can thank them for giving us a clue as to what this syndrome is all about.

It turns out we've known about this for 70 or 80 years and are learning more about *who* is affected and *how* we are affected. One thing for certain—this is real, and it has significant consequences. Those of us who bear this diagnosis have a significantly increased risk of developing cardiovascular disease (heart disease, strokes, and especially heart failure) and diabetes. Serious business, so how do I know if I have it?

Here's a list of five all-too-common medical conditions (all definitions are from the American Heart Association guidelines). If I have three of the five, I have the syndrome.

1. *Abdominal (central) obesity*—a waist circumference greater than 40 inches in men and 35 inches in women. Some

experts describe this as apple-shaped obesity, with adipose (fat) tissue accumulating mainly around the waist and trunk. We're not really sure why this is significant, but a clear connection exists between this type of obesity and the development of several types of heart disease as well as diabetes. While this definition uses waist circumference as the criterion, most experts also include a BMI of 30 or greater as a qualifier for this factor.

2. *Elevated blood pressure*—blood pressure equal to or greater than 130/85 or use of medication for hypertension. A couple of important points here. This threshold level is a little higher than what we'll be talking about as being normal, and may be changed in the near future. The other point is use of medication. More than a few of my patients have wrongly assumed that if they're taking blood pressure medicine, they no longer have hypertension. Nice try, but that's not the way it works. The same is true for those of us on medication for diabetes.

3. *Elevated fasting glucose*—equal to or greater than 100 mg/dl or use of medication for diabetes. Here again, an elevated blood sugar or treatment for diabetes satisfies this definition. Some experts would include those of us with *impaired glucose tolerance,* frequently called *pre-diabetes.*

4. *Elevated triglycerides*—equal to or greater than 150 mg/dl.

5. *Reduced HDL* (the good cholesterol)—less than 40 mg/dl in men and 50 in women.

It takes only three out of five of these to qualify for the metabolic syndrome, and one in three Americans has it. These conditions are very common and negatively impact our health and threaten our enjoyment of living.

The causes of this disorder seem intuitively obvious. Some are just that, but others are more perplexing. While the exact mechanisms of this complex condition are not fully known, several interconnecting pathways shed light on its causes. Let's take a look.

Obesity (especially central obesity). This is a key feature of the syndrome, and a body mass index (BMI) of 30 or greater should alert a person and their healthcare provider to this problem. We've already seen how being overweight is directly connected to heart disease, diabetes, and high blood pressure. Interestingly, since only three of the five medical conditions are required for the diagnosis, it is possible to be of normal weight and still have the syndrome, though we don't see this very often.

Stress. Surprised? This is complicated, and the association between the metabolic syndrome and stress is probably due to the effects of chronic stress on several hormonal activities in our brain. We know that stress increases cortisol levels (one of the stress hormones), which in turn raises glucose and insulin levels, increasing all the bad things they can do. This may help explain the connection between psychosocial stress and the development of heart disease.

Sedentary lifestyle. Just what you would expect. Less physical activity is directly related to heart attacks and strokes, as well as to the development of diabetes. Many components of the metabolic syndrome are clearly associated with an inactive lifestyle. These include a reduced HDL, increased blood pressure and blood sugar, and obesity. We'll consider what constitutes a sedentary lifestyle a little later and look at appropriate types, levels, and duration of various physical activities.

Aging. Unfortunately, we're all a little older since we started this chapter. Not much to do about this, except be aware that the incidence of this syndrome increases with increasing age. The number begins to approach one out of every two of us as we pass the 50-year mark. And more women than men are afflicted with the metabolic syndrome.

Diabetes. In addition to being one of the defining factors of this disorder, it seems the syndrome itself increases the likelihood of developing type 2 diabetes. We're not sure which is the cart and which is the horse here, but the two are clearly connected. The same appears to be true for coronary heart disease.

So, we know the importance of this problem, how to diagnose it, and some of the things that cause it. Now, how do we fix it?

The cornerstone of treatment is an honest appraisal of our lifestyle, identifying problems, and then making appropriate changes. Sounds simple enough, but as a physician (and sometimes a patient), I can readily tell you it is not. Those changes will probably include increased levels of exercise, a proper diet (a significant reduction in carbohydrate intake is critically important here), adequate sleep, stress reduction (again, easier said than done), and carefully targeted medication. This is a challenging issue to manage, and one that needs to be attacked on a multitude of fronts. While daunting, it can be done.

When it comes to medication, knowing where to start can be tricky, and it requires some expertise on the part of your healthcare provider. Most of us—patients and physicians alike—want to jump in and get started *right now*. "Don't just stand there, *do* something!" The correct approach, as with many things in life, may in fact be "Don't just do something, stand there." Or at least give some thought to your plan of action.

This is certainly true for dealing with the metabolic syndrome. We start with basic lifestyle changes, and then begin to attack specific problems with appropriately selected medications—sort of like a jigsaw puzzle. We start with the edges—something we can readily identify—and then look for other recognizable pieces. Pretty soon, the puzzle begins to make sense and things come together.

It's important to remember that we didn't develop the syndrome overnight, and it's not going to suddenly and magically go away. It takes a lot of work and effort on the part of the individual and a lot of support and guidance from our physician. But the results will be worth it—better control of our blood pressure, better control of our diabetes (maybe even eliminating the need for medication for these two conditions), better control of our weight, and less risk of a stroke or heart attack.

Who wouldn't want that?

7

A Brief History of Weight Loss

Our earliest predecessors didn't have much time to sit around glued to their iPads or laptops. They were busy hunting and gathering. Finding something to eat and surviving were top items on their agendas, and we probably wouldn't have found many, if any, tubby cave dwellers.

Things began to change as we became more civilized and began to exercise our dominion over creation. We learned how to farm, and raise and maintain herds of animals. And once we perfected the cultivation of wheat, the battle of the bulge was on.

This didn't happen in the 1950s or '60s but thousands of years ago. And some of our earliest writers and physicians seemed to be aware of the dangers of obesity. Hippocrates, the father of Western medicine, believed that in addition to being a problem in and of itself, being overweight ushered in a whole host of other medical problems. He was right, of course, as were the ancient Greeks and Egyptians before him. Once we mastered the production of food, we faced the challenge of consuming too much of it. For a while though, and as recently as a few hundred years ago, having a substantial girth was associated with being successful and well-to-do. A size 50 belt was a status symbol. Consider the portraits of Henry the Eighth. He was a big boy, and he proudly displayed his royal rotundity. Worked for him—but not so much for his wives.

More recently in our own country, most of us have seen pictures of William Howard Taft, the twenty-seventh president of the United States.

He was certainly not a model of fitness, and the story goes that on at least one occasion he became stuck in his bathtub. While that may or may not be true, he was known to frequently cause it to overflow. Taft might well have been a poster child for obesity and weight loss. He was the heaviest of all US presidents (sporting a BMI of more than 48!) and suffered from the things we would expect. He had significant hypertension (a systolic pressure of greater than 200); he frequently fell asleep during meetings, at meals, and even while standing; and he developed heart disease (suffering several heart attacks during his later years). Yet after leaving office, he lost more than 80 pounds, with many of his health problems improving.

Our attitudes and perceptions of obesity have gradually evolved in this country, with the growing understanding that being overweight is the cause of many of our physical maladies. But as with most pendulums, we need to be on guard for it swinging too far.

It seems that between the years 1922 and 1999, the average height of Miss America pageant *winners* increased by 2 percent, while the average weight decreased by 12 percent. There are fine lines between healthy and slim and skinny, as evidenced by the increasing prevalence of eating disorders in this country. We'll need to look at that later.

In spite of this change in our way of thinking about weight, over the past few decades we have experienced an ever-increasing prevalence of obesity in this country. Something is not matching up. We see being slender as something to be desired, something healthy, and yet we continue to fail in the goal of making that happen. This is a complex problem, as we've already seen, and we'll be considering many of these factors later on. But one thing is clear: Most of us want to weigh less than we do today. That brings us to a big step in the history of weight loss—the evolution of the weight-loss industry. And make no mistake about it, this is a huge industry.

We spend billions of dollars each year in our quest to lose weight. Since you're reading this book, you must have some desire to trim off a few pounds, maybe more. And since you're reading this book, you haven't yet discovered the long-sought-for secret method or the magical pill that ensures a perfect weight. If there were such things, there would be no need for this book and no global epidemic of obesity with its attendant maladies. But alas, there is no magic bullet, only hard work, dedication, and discipline. Since these attributes seem to be in short supply, a robust and ever-growing weight-loss industry has stepped in to entice us with promises of quick and easy fixes. Let's consider a few of the more imaginative offerings.

Several fad diets were developed prior to the 1900s, including a couple of low-carb approaches (which would ultimately prove to be on the right track), a diet that stressed flattened potatoes and vinegar, various forms and schedules of fasting, and all-liquid diets. But it wasn't until the turn of the twentieth century that things really became interesting.

One particular approach—the chewing diet—became popular in the early 1900s. It was simple: You could eat as much as you wanted but had to chew each mouthful at least 100 times. I suppose the theory was that eventually your jaw muscles would get tired, your wife had cleared the table after two hours, or you simply gave up. Legend has it that John D. Rockefeller and John Harvey Kellogg (of Tony the Tiger fame) were fans.

Then we're told of a parasite diet. If you were slender as a child, someone somewhere probably told you, "You're so skinny, you must have a tapeworm." Parasitic infections (tapeworms, hookworms, all kinds of worms) are associated with weight loss, among other things. If you could induce a tapeworm infection, you should be able to induce weight loss. Apparently you could buy capsules that contained the eggs of these worms, take a couple, and watch the pounds melt away. Sounds a little drastic to me, and if you've ever seen a microscopic picture of a tapeworm, you would and should find it repulsive. Probably wasn't FDA approved.

The nicotine diet, or more specifically the cigarette diet, came into vogue during the 1920s and '30s. The tobacco industry realized that smokers didn't weigh as much as nonsmokers and touted their products as being significant weight-loss tools. We know how that ended.

An interesting piece of weight-loss history has to do with the introduction of the calorie as a measure of the energy content of food. This happened in 1918 and forever changed how we view food, weight loss, and the cosmos. Everything we eat has an attached *calorie content*, and this simple unit has defined our approach to food and dieting. As an example, healthcare providers have been using American Diabetes Association (ADA) diets for decades—1000 calories, 1200 calories, 1500, and so on. This has been useful and effective. At the same time, we've become obsessed with the calorie, constantly seeking the lowest-calorie foods, snacks, and beverages possible. It all has to do with a balanced approach, and understanding that things go bad with the extremes. We'll be looking at how calories fit into a sensible weight-loss program later on.

Following the advent of the calorie, various specialized diets become popular. Some of these included the cabbage soup diet (pretty much what you'd expect), the Beverly Hills diet (stressing the "correct" order in which to eat our meals and a lot of pineapple), and an interesting blood-type diet. The theory with this approach assumed that each specific blood type (A, O, AB, and so on) should follow a specific kind of diet, with varying amounts of protein/carbohydrates, depending on the type. This makes a lot of sense. I mean really, when was the last time you saw an overweight vampire?

And then we have a long and fascinating list of physical approaches to weight loss. These include the use of a tiny fork, potentially limiting the amount of food you can eat at one sitting (chopsticks do that for me), multiple contraptions that vibrate various parts of your body (I suppose to shake off the fat), electrical stimulation of large muscles (lose weight while eating chips and watching TV), and a multitude of fat-melting creams and toning gels (all working while you sleep). The advent of television ushered in a whole new avenue for selling this stuff, and the Internet caused this cottage industry to explode. You can't surf more than a few pages without coming upon a new and painless way to get the body you've always wanted in two and a half weeks.

Lastly, we need to mention fasting. This idea has been around for centuries—actually millennia—usually within a spiritual context. Multiple examples are given us in the Bible of the need and benefits of fasting. In the context of weight loss, things are a little different. It makes sense that if you don't eat, you're going to lose weight. And that's what happens—unless you gorge yourself on the nonfasting days. Most fasting diets recommend a 5:2 ratio—five days of sensible eating and two days of fasting. Hard to do, and not necessarily healthy. But it will work. The issue of course is sustainability—can I do this for the rest of my life?

Probably not, and that's where the help in this book comes in. We're going to find ways to change our lifestyles, take a close look at what we're eating, lose some weight, and then have a plan to keep it off. Too good to be true? Nope. But we need to know where we're headed, and we need to have a goal. And don't worry. It won't include any tapeworms, blood-typing, or excessive cabbage.

Setting a Goal

If you don't know where you're going, you'll end up somewhere else.

Yogi Berra

With any journey, you should probably know where you're heading before you start out. That turns out to be true when we embark on a weight-loss plan. What's our goal? Do we have one? Do we even need one?

Remember, more than 60 percent of Americans are trying to lose weight. But most of us in this group aren't doing the things necessary to be successful—proper diet, exercise, and other lifestyle changes. And most don't have a realistic goal for their weight loss even though experts tell us that having such a target is critical if we're going to be successful. So yes, we do need to set a goal.

This should be easy, right? Let's say I want to lose 20 or 25 pounds. I'll simply write my target weight on a piece of paper and tape it to the refrigerator door. That should be a motivator, right?

Wrong.

The key component in setting a weight-loss goal is that it needs to be realistic. If not, we're almost certainly doomed to failure. But what is realistic? Why is it not reasonable to set an aggressive target and get started?

Physicians who are experienced in dealing with weight loss—especially with successful weight loss—tell us that most people don't have a realistic goal when asked about a desired target. When pressed for a number, a 20 to 30 percent reduction from their current weight is the usual response.

Let's think about that for a moment. If you're a 190-pound man, that 30 percent goal would mean you would need to lose 57 pounds! That's not going to happen. Even a 20 percent reduction would be 38 pounds.

If you're a 150-pound woman, a 20 percent reduction target would be 30 pounds. Not realistic, is it? Yet most of us have these kinds of numbers in mind, whether we realize it or not. And the vast majority of us will never achieve that degree of weight loss. We fail, become discouraged, and quickly regain whatever weight we might have lost.

So, what's a realistic number? How are we to determine a reasonable goal for our weight loss? For most of us, a 5 to 7 percent reduction is a sensible and practical goal. That would require significant and consistent lifestyle changes. If we add carefully considered drug and behavioral interventions, that target could become 10 to 15 percent. So let's pick a number of 8 to 10 percent. That should be achievable for most of us. That 190-pound man would write down a number of 15 or so pounds. And the woman—a 10- to 12-pound weight loss would be a realistic goal. If these two individuals achieve their targets, our experts would call this a good to excellent outcome.

Doesn't sound too difficult, does it? Not like that 57-pound number. With those goals in mind, what's our time frame? What's a reasonable period to have in mind for this loss? After all, that's part of our goal setting too. Once again, we have to be realistic. Weight loss of 8 to 10 percent can happen over six to eight weeks. A loss of one or two pounds a week is reasonable and achievable. That's the important point here. If we set realistic goals for ourselves—something meaningful that will improve our health and the way we feel about ourselves—we can get there.

So set your goal, write it down somewhere, and put your plan into action.

Getting It Right

Jakey Taylor

The transformation was startling. Jakey Taylor looked 10 years younger than his chronological age of 50. I sat down in front of his exam table and stared at him.

"How long has it been, Dr. Lesslie? A year and a half? Maybe two? I know I haven't been very diligent in coming in for my routine checkups."

I first met Jakey 15 years earlier. He was an executive with a large manufacturing company in town and had been a walking time bomb. High blood pressure, elevated cholesterol, two-pack-a-day smoking habit, and at least 30 extra pounds.

None of my admonitions for improving his health phased him. Not the risk of a heart attack or stroke, and not even his looming absence from the lives of his wife and three college-aged sons. Jakey was focused on his career and providing for his family.

"I'll have time later on to work on my health," he had said more than once. "Right now, though, I just need to keep taking those pills for my blood pressure and cholesterol. And hey, can you write me a prescription for a year's worth this time? I won't have to rearrange my schedule every couple of months, and that'll make it easier on me."

Knowing Jakey back then, I knew we were lucky to be getting him in the office once a year, if that. But each visit would give me another opportunity to try to impress upon him the dangerous path he was on and the serious consequences that inevitably awaited. We did make some progress several years ago with his smoking. He managed to cut down to one pack a day, but that happened more from his anger with the rising price of cigarettes than from a conviction that these things were killing him. Yet it was a victory—a step in the right direction.

Then we lost touch with him. I flipped through his record, looking for the date of the last visit.

"Two and a half years, Jakey," I told him. "That was the last time you were here."

"Wow, that long?"

"Uh-huh. Tell me how you've been doing. You look great."

Today he weighed 35 pounds less than he did on that last office visit. He was trim and healthy-looking, and I didn't see a bulge in his shirt pocket.

His eyes followed mine and he tapped the long-time residing place of his Marlboros. "Gave up the cigarettes a year ago. Stopped cold turkey, and boy was that hard. But I'll never pick them up again. What a filthy habit, and it was breaking me down. Just like you said it would."

"Tell me about your weight loss. Thirty-five pounds is a lot. How did you do it?"

Jakey smiled and leaned forward. "That was hard too, Dr. Lesslie. But once I got motivated, it just started happening. I remembered your advice about the low-carb diet and I bought a couple of books about it. Took a while to convince my wife it was the thing to do, but I finally managed to get her to try it, and she's lost 22 pounds. It's a lot easier when both of us are doing the same thing. We can help and encourage each other. She's a big reason I've been able to lose that weight. Her and the boys."

"So you finally decided you wanted to be around for their college graduation and for your grandchildren."

"That, sure. But it was something even more basic. It was a weekend trip on the Appalachian Trail."

"That sounds interesting. Tell me about it." I leaned back against the counter and closed his chart.

"About a year and a half ago, the boys wanted to go on a backpacking trip up in the mountains. They've always been active and into all kinds of sports. It didn't even occur to me that I'd have any trouble keeping up with them, but they taught me a thing or two. We borrowed a couple of tents and equipment and headed up toward the Asheville area.

"Beautiful place to hike, if you've never done it before. We got there Friday evening and headed out, hiking for an hour or so before we pitched camp. That wasn't too bad, and I did fine. Wasn't too tired. But in the morning, I was stiff and sore all over and could barely get out of the tent. We fixed some breakfast, and the boys were packed and ready to go while I was looking for the nearest exit. But I was stuck. We had committed, and that was that. We hiked all day and finally stopped and pitched camp again. I could barely move. My knees were killing me, and I was huffing and puffing like some old geezer. The boys were afraid I was going to have a heart attack or something. So was I.

"That night, I was just praying I'd be able to make it down the mountain and home in one piece. Thankfully we did, and that Sunday night after I crawled into bed, I told my wife something had to change. The extra weight I was carrying around was wearing out my knees and back. And I knew the cigarettes were ruining my lungs. I've never been so short of breath in all my life. I'll tell you, Doc, I never want to feel that way again."

"And that's when you started your diet."

"That's right," he answered. "I picked up those books I told you about, read everything I could about the low-carb thing, and we got started. I bought a treadmill and some free weights. That's been something we've all been able to do together, and that helps a lot. And you know what? Since I've lost the weight, my knees don't hurt anymore, and I don't get short of breath. Not even when I'm jogging on that treadmill."

"Good for you, Jakey. I'm really proud of you. None of this is easy to do, but you've found the key. It's having the motivation to get started and keep going."

He grinned at me and said, "And a couple of weeks ago, we went on another weekend backpacking trip. Those boys of mine—they ate my dust the whole way."

Let's Get Started!

Okay, it's time to organize a plan and put it into action. After all, "every long journey begins with a single step," and "there's nothin' to it but to do it"…or something like that. And the first and most important step? Believing that we're going to be successful. We're going to set a reasonable goal and we're going to get there. Yes, we're going to get there.

If you haven't decided on a goal yet, go back a few chapters, read why this is so important, and write down a target. You absolutely have to know where you're headed, and you absolutely have to know where you are. What's your BMI? Is it already ideal? Or are you in the overweight or obese zones? Maybe in one of the gray areas? You've got to know this because it will inform you as to your risk factors, the approaches that will probably work, those that won't, and even where to start with your plan.

Got it? Write your weight and BMI number down somewhere and we'll get going. And write down your goal. Remember, a loss of 5 to 7 percent of your initial body weight by the end of six weeks would be a great result. If you need to lose more than that, this would be a huge first step.

So what are our options? As with any health-related concern, we're always going to start with an honest evaluation of our lifestyle. This will include the sexy and exciting combination of diet, exercise, and behavioral modification. Well, maybe not sexy, but this evaluation will prove to be the cornerstone of any successful weight-loss plan. Experts tell us that lifestyle changes alone can result in an initial loss of that 5 to 7 percent (around ten pounds for the average American woman).

So what do we mean by "lifestyle changes"? And how hard can that really be? Let's start with changing how we talk about this and use the term "comprehensive lifestyle program." And it does need to be *comprehensive.* This must involve the important areas of our lifestyles, and in order for this to really work, it needs to be a program. The good news is that we won't have to plow new dirt. The Diabetes Prevention Program (DPP) has already outlined the important components of this, and these guidelines can be easily found on the Internet.

As we consider this, we'll quickly see that the foundation of a successful weight-loss effort includes *behavioral modification.* This involves the ability to make long-term changes in our eating patterns and consistently exercising our bodies. We're going to consider all of these facets in detail as we journey together through this book, but for now we need to have an understanding of what a good weight-loss program looks like. And changing our behavior is an important part of that. It's also a difficult part not easily achieved on our own. Most experts in this field tell us this usually requires the help of trained personnel, whether they be psychologists, physical trainers, or group counselors. Just as we find with giving up smoking, it's hard to do this on our own, and having someone helping and pulling for us is a good thing. It doesn't have to be in someone's office or clinic, though, and the Internet has some excellent sites that will help us. Here are a couple of examples:

- Christy Matta, "5 Cognitive Behavioral Strategies for Losing Weight that Work," *PsychCentral* (www.psychcentral.com/ blog/archives/2013/09/18/5-cognitive-behavioral-strategies -for-losing-weight-that-work/)

- "Cognitive Behavioural Therapy for Weight Loss (CBT)," *Virtual Medical Centre* (www.myvmc.com/treatments/ cognitive-behavioural-therapy-for-weight-loss-cbt/)

This idea of changing our behavior is important, and something we need to incorporate into our program. Experience teaches that most of us will need some help.

Then we have the components of *diet* and *exercise*. We'll start with the diet part, understanding that the greatest (and most sustainable) weight loss occurs through programs that involve caloric restriction rather than those that stress increased energy expenditure through exercise. Both are important, but the latest information gives the thumbs-up to decreased calorie consumption. That's important and may explain why some of us never seem to get off the block or quickly reach a plateau in our weight loss. We have to burn up more energy than we're taking in (a negative energy balance).

And speaking of calories, here's a question to consider: If an average-sized adult spends all their time in bed each day, how many calories will they need to maintain their current weight? In other words, if you didn't move around at all, how many calories a day (how much energy) does your body need to keep all systems working?

1. 100 calories
2. 250 calories
3. 1000 calories
4. 2500 calories

This turns out be to an important concept, since this baseline number represents a benchmark, the lowest denominator of calories that we need to survive. The answer is 1000 calories—but that's only if we don't move around at all. If we're of average size, don't confine ourselves to bed (or the sofa), and consume somewhere between 800 and 1200 calories each day, we're going to lose weight. That's a universal truth. If one of my patients insists they're sticking to a 1200-calorie diet and just can't seem to lose any weight, they're not counting all their calories. Period. More about that when we talk about the importance of a food diary. For now, we need to keep this concept of energy balance, and the importance of our dietary choices and plan, firmly fixed in our minds.

Next is exercise. If you breathed a sigh of relief as you read the last section—the part where lowering your energy intake through diet turns out to be more effective than increasing your exercise level—that's okay. Losing those ten (or more) pounds doesn't have to include hours in the gym, on the road, or pumping iron. We need to move our bodies and exercise our muscles and heart, but moderation will get the job done. But just what do we mean by moderation?

The people who really know this stuff will tell us that each of us needs 150 minutes each week of relatively strenuous exercise—a little more than 20 minutes each day. This can be satisfied by sustained brisk walking—getting your heart rate up and breathing hard. Jogging, swimming, and biking will get it done too, but brisk walking has a lot of benefits. In the chapters on exercise, we'll see that there are many ways to achieve this goal of 150 minutes of exercise a week, and that there's something out there for each of us, no matter our physical limitations.

One important caveat, something I'm faced with almost daily:

"Doc, I get plenty of exercise at work. I'm walking all over the plant and doin' all kinds of stuff. Besides, I don't have time to do anything else when I get home. And anyway, I'm always too tired."

If we don't have 20 minutes to walk with our spouse or grandchild, or just ourselves to reflect on the happenings of the day, then we're too busy. And the guidelines for 150 minutes a week are for "leisure time," not taking into account anything that happens at work. That's another important point: This physical activity needs to be set aside specifically for that purpose.

All right, so we've briefly considered behavior modification, diet, and exercise. For most of us, if we take these things seriously and make some changes, we can lose weight and achieve our goal. The "most of us" would be those with a BMI under 30. If that number is greater than 30, we'll need to incorporate all of these things into our weight-loss program and will more than likely need to add some form of drug therapy. There are several safe and effective medications to choose from, and we'll be taking a close look at these. But as an accepted guideline, we won't be reaching for these drugs unless a person's BMI is more than 30, though most physicians will lower that number to 27 in the presence of *comorbidities* or simultaneous medical conditions such as diabetes and heart disease, where aggressive weight loss is something to be desired.

What if a person's BMI is greater than 40 (or more than 35 with some of those same comorbidities)? That's when we'll try the lifestyle changes, medications, and begin considering bariatric surgery. Most of us with a number greater than 40 won't be able to succeed in losing a meaningful amount of weight without significant help. Fortunately, it's out there and it's safe. But only in the right circumstances and in the right hands.

So that's how we're going to get started. You need to know your BMI and where you are in this spectrum of weight and weight-loss strategies. And you need to get going.

11

Keeping a Food Journal

Don't think this is important? Well, consider this: Those of us who keep an accurate food diary lose twice as much weight as those who don't. And those who do have a much better chance of keeping it off. That should be enough to get our attention.

The experts have known for quite a while that writing down what we eat is a simple and proven way to enhance our weight-loss efforts. Some think it is indispensable. It allows us to study our eating habits, identify problem areas and correct them, and monitor our progress. Sound simple? It is, but we need to keep some things in mind before we grab a pen and notebook.

The first thing is the notebook itself. This will work fine for a lot of us, but others might be more interested and consistent in using one of many apps available for our smartphones or even a laptop. A couple of good places to start are www.myfooddiary.com, www.mynetdiary.com/iPhone .html, and www.myfitnesspal.com. The point is to get organized and get started.

What does a food journal or diary need to look like? This is important, and we need to start off on the right foot—not having to backtrack and add information we should have been keeping right off the bat.

The first thing needs to be the *date*. See, I told you this was simple.

Then we need to note the *time of day*. This needs to be specific, since it will allow us to examine patterns in our eating habits.

Next should be the *location* where we're eating. Home, at the office, in a restaurant, in a car...these are all significant, but we also need to note the place we eat in our homes. Is this always the kitchen or dining area? What about in bed or in the playroom? Write it down. Again, we're looking for trends.

In this same context, we should note *who we're eating with or whether we're alone*. This is especially helpful if we have trouble binge eating and wonder when, where, and with whom it's happening.

The next two areas to record might not seem obvious, but they turn out to be critical as we try to understand how and why we eat. Make a note of *what you're doing while eating*, whether it's a sit-down meal with friends, at your computer while working on a book—excuse me while I take a bite of this chicken salad—watching TV in bed, or even talking on the phone. And note *the mood you're in*. Yes, your mood. Are you happy, tired, anxious, angry, or just so-so? Write it down. Not only will it help establish patterns of eating, but it will allow you to get more in touch with your feelings and emotions—a skill that many of us lack.

Also *consider whether you're actually hungry or not*, and make a note. This might surprise us as well, but we'll find that most of our eating is based on habits and not actual need. As part of this "mood analysis," keep space in your journal to note how you feel *after* eating. Why would we do this? Wouldn't it be helpful to remember how that microwaved plate of lasagna at midnight made us feel? Or how we felt after that third trip to the buffet table? Write it down and refer back to it. Insightful and motivating.

Now we get to the meat of the journal, and maybe the vegetables. Note *what you eat* and *how much of it*. The "how much" is just as important as the "what." Over time, we'll learn how to closely estimate our portion sizes, but at first we might need some help. Those three websites noted above will give us some help with this as well. This is where we have to be accurate and truthful. We must record *everything* we eat and drink. The drinking part is frequently where my patients go astray. They fail to write down the three glasses of sweetened iced tea or the two sodas. Those empty calories quickly add up and ruin your hard work.

This point really can't be stressed too much. In order for this journaling business to work, we have to be completely honest with ourselves and write down every single thing that passes our lips. Period.

Okay, so there are the things we need to be keeping track of. Now for some tips to help you be successful.

- Write down *everything* you eat. Didn't I just say that? Well, it's that important.

- Learn to estimate the amount of food you're eating—cups, ounces, even sizes (inches, if need be).

- Do your diary-keeping as soon as you can after eating. Our memories quickly fail, and things slip away. Make your notes throughout the day.

- Learn to be specific. Did you put cheese on your broccoli? How much? Gravy on your potatoes? (I hope you're not eating this.) If so, what kind of gravy and how much? You don't have to go overboard, but you need to be detailed enough to get an accurate picture of where your calories are coming from. A recent example from one of my patients is illustrative. His lunchtime meal included a diet soda and a ham-and-cheese sandwich. That was all that was written in his log. By the time he described this "simple" sandwich, we determined that it contained more than 800 calories. Quite a load. So be specific in your descriptions.

Now for a couple of common pitfalls. We already discussed a few of these, but they are common traps that can quickly ruin your weight-loss program.

- Make sure you include the beverages you consume. We find a lot of hidden calories here.

- Don't dismiss the emotional side of eating. Write down how you feel before and after eating. Were you driven to that chocolate cake by an argument with your spouse? Do home-budget worries send you to the fridge? And what about the uncomfortable guilt of that midnight pint of ice cream?

- Don't limit yourself to pen and paper. Consider one of the online apps and use it. Most of us are never far from our smartphones or other electronic devices.

- Even though you document everything you eat, don't forget to be accurate in recording the size of your portions and the amounts of your servings.

That's about it. At the end of the day, or the end of the week, you'll have a good record of what you're eating. That's the time to reflect a little, study it for trends and patterns, and begin to make some changes. You won't need to do this forever—maybe only a few weeks. You'll know when you've learned enough and can set the journal aside for a while. But don't throw it away. Most importantly, remember that this journal is your friend, something to be appreciated for what it can help you do—lose weight.

12

What's This Waist-Hip Ratio Business?

Comparing Apples to Pears

A pound is a pound is a pound. Right? Not so fast. It turns out that how and where we add those extra pounds says a lot about our overall health. This all has to do with *body composition*, something we've known about for quite a while, but we have struggled with how to make it applicable to the assessment and management of obesity and the improvement of our health. Let's start with some basic science.

Each of us is composed of a handful of atomic building blocks: oxygen (61 percent of our total weight), carbon (23 percent), hydrogen (10 percent), nitrogen (2.6 percent), calcium (1.4 percent), and around 1 percent of an assortment of other atoms (potassium, sodium, chlorine, phosphorus, magnesium, and several trace elements). These atoms are then combined into various molecules (more than 100,000 of them), ranging from the very simple (water) to the very complex (long strands of DNA and specialized proteins). Of these molecules, water makes up at least 60 percent of a man's weight (a little less for a woman), protein comprises 15 percent of normal body composition, minerals (calcium, magnesium, and so on) 5 percent, with body fat making up the rest (as little as 10 percent in well-trained athletes and up to 50 percent in those of us who are markedly obese).

It's the fat content of our bodies that we're interested in, since this is where we store excess energy and what we want to eliminate in our weight-loss efforts. But where do we store this excess fat?

Most of us are probably looking down at our bellies at this point, and that would be a logical assumption. But it would be wrong. The majority of our body fat (up to 80 percent in men and 90 percent in women) is found in our *subcutaneous tissues* (*sub*: "under"; *cutaneous*: "skin"), thus effectively distributed just under the surface of our entire bodies. This is easy to see and feel.

There's another type of body fat—called *visceral adipose tissue*—that we don't see and that we need to be more concerned about. This fat is deposited around our abdominal organs (liver, pancreas, stomach, intestines), and when its amount is increased, we see a much greater risk of high blood pressure, heart disease, and diabetes. But if we can't see it, how do we determine if we have too much of it?

That's the important question, and it's what experts in this area have struggled with. There are complex (and expensive) ways to analyze the percentage of body fat in an individual, such as using elaborate X-ray studies or submersion in a specialized tub of water. But we need something simple and safe to give us an idea of the magnitude of our personal problem, or to determine if we in fact have one. Fortunately for us, such a technique exists.

This a good time to mention *impedance measurement*, because that's not it. You might have had this done in your doctor's office, weight-loss center, or company-sponsored health fair. It involves the application of electrodes to one arm and one leg, squeezing the grips of a small handheld device, or standing on the foot plates of a specialized scale. The impedance of an imperceptible electrical current is measured across two points, indicating the amount of resistance between those electrodes. From this measurement, a calculation is made to determine your percentage of body fat. These are calculations, and they amount to an estimation only. There are several potential sources of error with these devices, and individual results vary too much to make this useful. Interesting, but not accurate.

So let's get back to this simple and safe technique. All we'll need is a nonstretchable tape measure, with inches on one side and centimeters on the other. That's it. Nothing more elaborate. But this turns out to be an important tool for each of us.

This is one place where it's not appropriate to compare apples to apples. On the contrary, we want to compare apples to pears. Let's start with the pears.

The title of this chapter provides the needed insight here—we're going to compare our waist size to our hip size. And it's really very simple. If our hips are larger than our waist, we fall into the category of being shaped like a pear. That's a good thing, since this type of fat storage is associated with having less visceral fat (the bad kind). On the other hand, if the circumference of our waist is larger than our hips, we're an apple and will have more visceral fat.

While making these measurements is not rocket science, there are right and wrong ways of doing it. Here's the correct way:

Stand with your feet close together, wearing little or no clothing. Relax as much as you can and exhale normally. At the end of this exhalation, take two measurements of your hips. If they're within one centimeter of each other, take an average and you have your number. If the difference is more than one centimeter, shake it off, assume the position again, and remeasure. The hips can be measured at their widest point or at the top of the iliac crests (the boney top of each side of the pelvis). Then repeat the process for your waist. The waist is best measured just *above* the belly button.

Once you have these numbers, divide the waist measurement by the hip measurement, giving you the waist-hip ratio (WHR). Most experts agree that for women, a ratio of greater than 0.8 is associated with an unhealthy distribution of body fat (increased heart disease, diabetes, high blood pressure) and for a man that number is 0.9. While there are other ways to determine body composition, the WHR is quick and easy, and it's the only one that takes into account our many body types.

From the standpoint of our weight-loss efforts, the WHR gives us a helpful (but perhaps troubling) piece of information, though we won't need to constantly be measuring this. What we *should* be measuring monthly is our waist circumference. This, along with our BMI, gives us a good idea of our progress. And along with our BMI, it gives us another goal or target to consider. Once again, we have to be realistic in our aspirations here. Few, if any, will achieve the pear shape and waistline of Scarlett O'Hara. But we need to strive to avoid the apple.

13

The Lowly Calorie

Unloved, Unappreciated, Yet So Important

Each one of us is familiar with the calorie, or at least we better be if we're going to plan and successfully execute a weight-loss effort. The word originates from the Latin root for "heat." As such, the calorie began its illustrative career in the chemistry and physics labs, where it became a precisely defined measure of energy. Technically, one calorie represents the amount of energy needed to raise the temperature of one gram of water by one degree (Celsius) at a specific barometric pressure. Sort of like "one horsepower," which is the amount of power it takes a healthy horse to raise 550 pounds one foot in one second. (That might come in handy someday if you're ever on *Jeopardy*.) For our purposes, we're interested in the calorie as a measure of the energy content of the food and beverages we consume.

In case you've ever been confused by the terms "calorie" and "kilocalorie," they represent different amounts of the same thing—a kilocalorie is 1000 calories. This differentiation is important if you're studying basic chemistry, but in regards to modern medicine and dietary planning, they are used interchangeably.

Now let's consider the energy content of our food, and why that's important. Each of our bodies is a virtual biochemical nuclear reactor. There's stuff going on every microsecond of every day. And when the reactor stops, we stop. Consider what's going on inside you as you read this page. Muscles are constantly contracting and relaxing while keeping us upright, cells throughout your body are being built up or destroyed and replaced, complex chemical processes are humming along, your heart is beating, and an elaborate system of checks and balances keeps your core temperature hovering around 98.6 degrees Fahrenheit.

All of these take energy—our *basal* (baseline) *metabolic rate* (BMR). And where does this energy come from? Right—the food we consume. Our digestive tract is remarkably capable of converting the things we eat and drink into usable fuel, which our body then burns to accomplish the tasks mentioned above. This BMR is important to understand. If we decide to take a day off and spend it in bed watching TV or reading, we're still going to be burning fuel for energy—a baseline amount. Our BMR is fairly constant, though it can change over time. (This is an important fact, as we'll learn when we discuss the plateau of weight loss, or "hitting the wall.") The BMR—our daily calorie requirement—is determined by such things as our age, gender, weight, and physical activity. This is where the math gets pretty simple. Our body will use only the amount of energy it needs to perform the tasks at hand, and it will derive this fuel from what we eat. If we take in more energy/fuel than we need, we convert the remainder to fat, store it away, and gain weight. If we take in less than we need, we find another source of energy (hopefully the excess stored fat) and burn that, thus losing weight.

So we have some baseline energy needs as well as the need for more fuel for any extra physical activity or other demands we may encounter. In terms of calories, what does this BMR look like? If you're a 30-year-old man and you get around 30 minutes of moderate exercise a day, your basic daily calorie needs will be around 2400. A 50-year-old male with the same amount of exercise will need a little less—around 2000 calories a day. For a 30- and then a 50-year-old woman (with the same amount of exercise), those numbers would be 2000 and 1600.

This gives us a general idea of the amount of fuel or energy we need to maintain our current weight. Take in more, we gain weight. Take in less, we lose it. That's why having an understanding of our calorie intake is so important if we're going to successfully lose weight. Most experts recommend a general target—usually in the range of 1500 calories per day—for effective weight loss. This could be more if you're physically very active or less if there are circumstances that prevent regular exercise. But 1500 calories is a commonly prescribed goal.

Now here's some information we need to keep tucked away somewhere: It takes about 3500 excess calories to pack on one pound of weight (we're talking about fat here). The converse is also true: It takes 3500 calories of excess physical activity or reduced food intake to lose that one pound. This is where life is just not fair. It's really easy to add those 3500 calories and gain that pound, but it becomes very difficult to do the opposite. Adding that pound takes only a few slices of pizza, a couple of plates of spaghetti, and a bowl or two of ice cream. But to burn up those same 3500 calories takes more than seven hours of brisk walking. Seven hours! It's just not fair.

(For an interesting source of information for where those calories come from, check out www.calorielab.com.)

Now we need to clear up some more potential confusion—the "empty calorie."

"Doc, I've read that a lot of things have empty calories in them. If they're empty, they shouldn't cause me to gain weight, right?"

Wrong.

A calorie is still a calorie and contains the same amount of energy-producing fuel. The problem with an empty calorie is that's all it contains—the energy but no significant nutrients, such as amino acids, fiber, vitamins, minerals, and antioxidants. Some examples of these would be foods with added sugars or solid fats, such as

- candy
- ice cream
- cookies or cake
- margarine and various shortenings
- added sugars (frequently high-fructose corn syrup)
- beer, wine, and other alcoholic beverages

We're not going to be able to avoid all of these empty calories, and a certain amount is going to be okay. For that 50-year-old man we considered earlier, up to 270 of these calories a day would not be a problem. And for that 50-year-old woman? Up to 160 empty calories would be accept-able. More than those amounts and we're adding on the calories but not achieving our nutritional goals. Something to keep in mind.

So there's the lowly calorie. It's your friend or foe, depending on how you put this information to use.

14

Exercise, Part 1

Ya Gotta Get Movin'

We hear it all the time: "Get up and do something!"

"Don't become a couch potato."

"Just do it."

We know we should be exercising, but sometimes it's hard to get started. Where do we find the motivation for that first step or first sit-up or first push-up? Maybe we need to start with the *why*, and then figure out the *how*.

It turns out the *why* is pretty overwhelming. The list of the benefits of physical activity is long and sometimes surprising.

As we would expect, exercise protects against the development of many common chronic conditions—heart disease, diabetes, chronic lung disease, kidney disease, and some kinds of cancers. Some experts believe the risk of recurrent breast cancer can be lowered by as much as 50 percent and the risk of developing colon cancer reduced by up to 60 percent. Alzheimer's disease falls into this category as well—something that should get the attention of those of us in our middle years and beyond. And it should come as no surprise that physical activity reduces the incidence of obesity, with all the problems associated with being overweight.

Now here are a few surprising benefits. The risk of osteoporosis is reduced with weight-bearing exercise. Bone mineral density increases, which reduces the possibility of a hip or other type of fracture. And since physical activity improves muscle tone and balance, the chances of falling are significantly diminished.

Exercise also decreases the risk of gallstones as well as improving brain function (again, lowering the risk of several types of dementia, including Alzheimer's). Regular physical activity can reduce stress and help lessen anxiety and depression. We previously mentioned that vigorous exercise can help you get to sleep faster and can improve the quality of your sleep, making it deeper and more efficient.

When it comes to lipids (cholesterol levels), the benefits are important and straightforward. We know that regular exercise can lower LDL and triglyceride levels and raise HDL levels—all things we want to see happen.

With most of these benefits, the effect appears to be "dose-related"— the longer and more vigorous the exercise, the greater the improvements we experience in both physical and psychological well-being. But how much is enough, and what kinds of exercise are we talking about?

Without getting too complicated, it might be helpful to consider how exercise physiologists measure exercise levels. They use the term metabolic equivalent (MET) to compare various forms of physical activity. For instance, one MET equals the amount of oxygen an adult would consume while sitting at rest. Moderate physical activity (swimming, general housecleaning, using a push mower, leisurely biking, and walking briskly at three to five miles per hour) would fall in the three- to six-MET range. Vigorous activity would be those things performed at greater than six METs and include running, push-ups and pull-ups, and jumping rope (try *that* sometime if you really want a good workout).

So with those definitions in mind, what should be our goals? Here are a few suggestions and examples:

- Vigorous exercise of at least 20 minutes three times a week, combined with 30 minutes of moderate activity on most days, has been associated with a 50 percent reduced risk of death in men and women aged 50 to 71 years.

- Another option is to combine 150 minutes of moderate exercise with 75 minutes of vigorous exercise each week.

And for those of us who fall in the "overly compulsive" category, we can use METs to quantify our activity level. Solid experimental evidence indicates that expending 500 to 1000 METs a week is necessary to achieve "substantial health benefits" (which these researchers define as a significant reduction in the risk of premature death and breast cancer). This equates to 150 minutes of walking each week (at 3.3 METs per minute, that gives you about 500). If so inclined, you can do the rest of the math to reach 1000, combining various physical activities.

Measuring your heart rate, while sometimes helpful, is not necessary, thus saving us money on various monitors and contraptions. As we can see, the key factors are *time* and *intensity.*

"But Dr. Lesslie," someone might say, "I *am* a couch potato. Shouldn't I have my doctor check me over before I start an exercise program?"

That's a good question, and the answer is…maybe. But probably not. If you're in good health and don't have a history of a significant medical problem (heart disease, diabetes, uncontrolled high blood pressure), it's probably okay to get started. But do so gradually. Start slowly and build from there.

On the other hand, if you do fall into one of those problem categories, it will be a good idea to talk with your physician about how and when to begin. Be prepared though. If you ask ten doctors this question, you'll probably get eleven different answers.

If in doubt about the need for a medical evaluation before beginning a vigorous exercise program, a couple of questionnaires will help guide you. You can find these at www.ncwc.edu/files/AHA.pdf.

The main point here is pretty simple—we need to get moving and keep moving. Exercise has to be a part of any successful weight-loss program, and we need to approach it objectively and as enthusiastically as we can. We'll need to first determine how much exercise we're getting now and then decide what kinds of things and how much of them we need to be doing. Many times, this plus a little calorie restriction will get us kickstarted and on our way.

Oh—and it's never too late to start.

15

Exercise, Part 2

Overcoming the Yo-Yo

If you've ever tried to lose weight, then you know about the yo-yo effect. We lose some weight, then we gain some weight, then we lose some weight…It's a frustrating but common problem, and a frequent reason for giving up on our weight-loss efforts. But it can be overcome. First, though, what do we know about the yo-yo?

As we start to lose weight—either intentionally, as with a diet, or unintentionally, as with several disease processes or starvation—our bodies respond in a predictable way. It's all about survival and our body's amazing ability to slow down our metabolic rate, reduce energy consumption and need, and live a little longer. This is important if we're on a deserted island with nothing to eat. But if we're keeping a food diary, reducing our calories, and trying to lose weight, our own body is working against these efforts.

Here's the vicious cycle: We lose weight, our metabolism slows, our body burns muscle in preference to fat (resulting in a long-term reduction in our baseline metabolism), and when we inevitably stop our diet and resume what had once been our normal caloric intake, we gain the weight back (much quicker than we lost it). We've created a "positive" energy balance—too much fuel for what we need. When we try to lose that weight, we get the same results: weight loss followed by weight gain. And finally we give up. That's the yo-yo.

As we noted, this is a common problem, and if a weight-loss program focuses only on calorie restriction, that's what we're going to get—and then failure. The key to preventing the yo-yo? Exercise. It has to be a part of any successful and sustainable weight-loss plan. That sounds obvious, but we need to understand why this is so.

We mentioned that during starvation (or intentional weight loss), our body burns muscle before it burns fat. The first choice is always glucose or glycogen, since simple sugars are the quickest and easiest source of energy. But we don't have large stores of these on hand, and our bodies quickly turn elsewhere. If we're not exercising and trying to build muscle mass, whatever muscle we do have will gradually be cannibalized. At the same time, we'll be burning a little fat, but again, that's our last resource. Unfair, but true.

And while unfair, we can put this physiologic principle to good use. Our muscles can be thought of as energy dynamos. They require constant blood flow and are constantly consuming and producing energy. Fat, on the other hand (or hip), is inert. It just sits there, with little blood supply since nothing much is going on. So what we want to do is increase the amount of energy dynamos in our body. We want our muscles to be humming along and helping us maintain our weight and maybe even lose some of the excess.

In the previous chapter, we considered various forms of physical activity and how to gauge the amount of exercise we're getting. Brisk walking is a good and simple way to achieve the minimum of 150 minutes we need each week, but we need to be doing something else. Resistance training (lifting free weights or dumbbells) will help build muscle mass in our arms, shoulders, and back. We can also incorporate various machines to target our legs and thighs. This doesn't have to be excessive, and our goal shouldn't be to achieve the perfect beach body. We're just trying to convince our body to burn more fat for its needed energy and to help us lose weight.

So does this work? Or can I just get out my Weight Watchers point calculator, stay on the sofa, and see how things go?

Combining exercise with calorie restriction (or point counting) is much more effective than reduced food intake alone. And it's the best way to ensure maintenance of your weight loss over the long haul. In fact, it's going to be the only way to overcome the metabolic resetting that takes place with weight loss. This is how we can overcome the yo-yo—as well as defeat the plateau that also looms ahead of us. More about that a little later.

While exercise is one of the cornerstones of lifestyle management and change, it's not a panacea. You'll never achieve your weight-loss goals with exercise alone. Think not? Then consider a couple of points.

Remember what we said about the calorie. To lose one pound of body weight (hopefully fat) will require a net loss of about 3500 calories. If our diet remains constant, and we walk for about 15 minutes each day (burning around 100 calories), it will take us at least five weeks to lose that one pound. That's a lot of walking for just one pound. And that assumes a constant diet. What happens when we succumb to the temptation of a piece of pecan pie? Boom—500 calories! That's going to be a lot of walking—about one hour of moderate hill climbing with 30 pounds on our back. Get the picture? That's why it can be difficult, but not impossible, to lose weight.

Here are some things to keep in mind about exercise:

- It should be viewed as an indispensable part of the weight-loss process, combined with calorie restriction.

- It has its limits. We won't be able to lose weight with increased exercise alone, and we shouldn't fall into the trap of thinking, *I'll eat this pecan pie and just stay on the treadmill for a few more minutes.*

- It has significant upside potential. In addition to reducing our chances of developing diabetes, high blood pressure, and heart disease, it allows us to lose weight where we most want to see it disappear—around our midsection. This happens with just about every form of exercise and physical activity, not just sit-ups and abdominal crunches.

The important thing is to get started and get moving. If you have limitations in the types of exercise you can perform, or if walking is all you can safely do, that's fine. Our minimum, though, is 150 minutes a week, with 300 minutes being a challenging but rewarding goal. For those of us able to be more active, a good multicomponent program will include balance training, flexibility maneuvers (especially important for those of us over the age of 60), aerobic exercise, and resistance training. The key is to find something you enjoy doing and someone to do it with.

Oh…and get started! The yo-yo can be a thing of the past.

Okay, I've been at this for about a month, and I've lost two pounds. Well, actually closer to one, but at least it's something. At this rate, I might never get to my goal. I can't increase my exercising any more, and my bladder won't let me drink any more water. I've been preaching this for a long time, and I'm just going to have to break down and start keeping a food diary. We'll see.

16

Getting It Wrong

Sarah Hoffman

"Wasn't she just here a couple of weeks ago?"

Amy Connors, the ER secretary on duty, nodded toward room 3. She was right. I had recognized the 17-year-old as Lori Davidson rolled her past the nurses' station in the triage wheelchair.

"Uh-huh," I said, glancing down at her clipboard. "Nausea and vomiting then. Looks like the same thing today."

"She looks worse to me," Amy added. "Pale as a ghost, and those dark rings under her eyes…She got something bad goin' on?"

Sarah Hoffman's vital signs were okay. Blood pressure 90/62. Heart rate 102—fast for someone sitting in a wheelchair. No fever.

My eyes were drawn to something Lori had circled at the top of the chart. Sarah's weight was only 92 pounds. I flipped to her last visit—barely two weeks earlier. She had lost seven pounds since then.

"Hmm." I picked up the chart and headed around the counter on my way to room 3.

"What?" Amy asked. "What's the matter?"

"*Something's* going on," I said quietly. "We'll have to find out."

Lori had transferred Sarah to the stretcher and was spreading a hospital sheet over the young woman.

"Her mother is out in the business office," Lori said. "I'll bring her back when she's finished with the paperwork."

Sarah turned her head away and pulled the thin sheet up to her chin.

"She's been vomiting since yesterday," Lori continued. "Can't keep anything down. Right, Sarah?"

No response—then barely a nod of her head.

I pulled over a rolling stool, sat down, and rested Sarah's chart on my lap.

"Okay, Miss Hoffman, tell me what's been going on."

When I had glanced at the ER record of her last visit, I saw where I had written "vague history," followed by "nausea, vomiting, mother worried about dehydration." I don't make a note of a vague history very often, so something must have gotten my attention.

I looked at the young girl. Amy was right—Sarah Hoffman was pale. The word *emaciated* came to mind, and I wrote it on the chart.

The curtain was drawn open, and Sarah's mother walked into the room and over to the stretcher.

"Dr. Lesslie, I'm glad it's you on duty today. You saw Sarah the last time she was here, and she's started it again—the nausea and vomiting. She was better for a few days and seemed to be turning the corner, but now this." She nodded at her listless daughter. "She's gotten to the point where she can't keep anything down. We're worried to death about her."

Lori handed me a lab slip. She had gotten a routine urinalysis while Sarah had been in triage, as well as a pregnancy test. That was negative, but her urine was really concentrated, with a markedly elevated ketone level. She was dehydrated—dangerously so.

"Tell me about what's been going on at home," I asked. "Other than the vomiting. Does Sarah have any medical problems or recent travel? Anything unusual?"

Mrs. Hoffman shook her head. "No, nothing out of the ordinary. No travel or anything. She stays busy with her schoolwork and cheerleading. They're in the midst of tryouts, and this is really setting her back."

"She's lost some weight, according to the record here." I pointed to the number at the top of the chart. "Some of that might be due to dehydration, but is there anything else going on? Has Sarah been trying to eat?"

Her mother chuckled. "Good luck with that. She's never been a big eater, and now with the cheerleading and all, she's obsessed with losing a couple of pounds. We keep telling her that she's fine and even needs to gain some weight. But you know how teenagers are. She won't listen to her father and me."

"Sarah, tell me about that." I studied the girl's profile and noticed her rapid, shallow respirations. I had missed that when I walked into the room. In addition to being dehydrated, she probably was acidotic, with her electrolytes all out of kilter.

She didn't respond. I tossed the ER chart to the countertop, got up, and walked over to the edge of her stretcher.

Lori had stepped around to the other side and was pricking the girl's finger for a routine blood-sugar test. New-onset diabetes could be a possibility here, and if her blood sugar was sky-high, that would explain the vomiting, weight loss, and dehydration. But there hadn't been any sugar in her urine.

"Fifty-two." Lori glanced up at me, the glucose monitor still in her hand.

That was low—really low. *What was going on here?*

I took her hand and found the thready pulse at her wrist. Around 100 and regular—but weak.

"Does she take any medication?" I asked her mother.

"No, none. Like I said, she doesn't have any medical problems and has always been in good health."

My hand rested lightly on her sunken abdomen. She grimaced and pushed it away.

"Sarah, let the doctor examine you," her mother said. "He needs to find out what's going on."

Lori drew the sheet down. Sarah was wearing a sweat suit emblazoned with the name of one of the local high schools. I raised the top a little, just enough to expose her abdomen.

Her mother gasped. "What is that?"

In the middle of her abdomen, just above her belly button, was an angry, golf-ball-sized abscess. Sarah tried to cover it with her hands. Lori gently but firmly intercepted her. No wonder she had grimaced. It had to be painful.

"Over here." Lori nodded at the side of the girl's belly. Another abscess was brooding—not yet quite as large as the first.

We found three more before pulling down her sweatshirt and covering her again with the sheet.

"Sarah, why didn't you tell me?" her mother said.

The girl turned her head to the wall again, silent.

Before we had covered her up, I noticed several small skin pricks, scattered on her abdomen and not yet infected. "Tell me about any medicine in the house," I asked her mother. "Anything you may be taking…or your husband."

"I take something for my blood pressure, but that's all. And her father has diabetes, but nothing else. Why?"

"Does he use insulin?" I asked, glancing again at Sarah.

"Yes, he does. But…" Her eyes traveled quickly from mine to Lori's. "You don't think she's…Sarah, have you been using your father's insulin? But why would she do that? She's not diabetic and doesn't have…" Her head jerked around and our eyes met. "Could she have been giving herself insulin injections to try to lose weight? Is that why she's vomiting and staying so sick?"

I looked down at her daughter. Without a word Lori was already reaching for an IV setup.

We had our answer.

17

Discipline

A Muscle in Need of Exercise

"I never metaphor I didn't like." This chapter will be no exception.

There are truths that govern this universe, and among those is the unfortunate reality, "If you don't use it, you'll lose it." Consider that for a moment and try to find an exception. It's true about hard-won musical talent and ability. Without practice, a pianist's fingers grow rusty, and a guitarist loses her touch and feel for the frets. It's true about our spiritual lives as well. Without prayer, reading, meditation, and fellowship, this part of our being grows stale and listless. We lose touch with our Touchstone.

Now consider our physical bodies and the many muscles that allow us to move our heads, walk around, and even breathe. Without regular exercise, they wither and grow weak. Think not? If we take a well-conditioned athlete—a football player or weight lifter—and put him at complete bedrest for as little as one week, drastic changes take place. Muscle tone is lost as well as muscle mass. It doesn't take very long for even the ability to walk to be lost. Years of hard work gone in a matter of days. That's harsh, but it's reality.

The same is true for the elusive virtue of discipline. It can be viewed as a muscle just like any other, one that needs to be regularly exercised in order to develop and become strong. And then to stay strong. Many of us seem to be able to call on a deep reservoir of discipline—"keeping our noses to the grindstone," making difficult things happen. For most of us, though, developing discipline requires work, and it's seldom easy.

How about you? Are you disciplined? Possessed of self-control? You might find it interesting to test yourself a little. The many electronic and technical distractions of this time in our American culture will make this easy to do. Pick one—just one—time-robbing activity that you pursue on your smartphone or computer. It could be one of the hundreds of variations of solitaire or a game you play with friends. If you can't think of one, congratulations. You're in a much-admired minority. For the rest of us, choose one of those activities and determine to give it up for one week. Just a week. Sounds easy, but maybe not so much. It requires determination and discipline. Temptations abound, and lapses lie waiting in each quiet moment. You'll see.

The connection between this kind of discipline and successful weight loss becomes apparent as we begin our journey. Choosing a diet and sticking with it, limiting our portion sizes, keeping an accurate diary, and exercising each day. All of these require discipline. Without it, we won't win our battle with our weight and with few of the other challenges we'll face as we travel through this life. But just like any other muscle, with attention and exercise, discipline will grow and become stronger. A little each day. One successful day becomes two, then three, then a week, and then a month. Just like giving up your game of solitaire.

Discipline is the bridge between goals and accomplishment.
Jim Rohn (1930–2009)

18

Water, Water Everywhere...

Since this is a book about weight loss and dieting…how long do you think you can live without food? If your answer is four to six weeks, you're right. Of course it all depends on a person's age and general health, but a month to a month and a half seems to be about the limit. Not the best way to plan your weight loss though.

How about water? Two days? Two weeks? Two months? The answer is about one week. Water is obviously very important to the human body, and it provides as much as 60 percent of our total body weight.

But what else does water do for us? Water is important in the functions of digestion, circulation, transportation of important nutrients, temperature regulation, and the efficient performance of all our vital organs. Plain and simple—we just can't live without it.

Water does other things for us that might not be as obvious. Adequate hydration can keep your skin looking good—something important for a lot of us. And it helps with exercise and muscle functioning. Without adequate hydration, our muscles just don't work as well as they should. Our exercise workouts don't go as well as we want, and at the extreme, progressive weakness can lead to imbalance and dangerous falls.

When it comes to maintaining or losing weight, adequate water intake is essential. This works in a couple of ways. By substituting plain water for beverages that contain sugar or other sources of calories, we reduce our overall calorie intake. And drinking water before and with a meal reduces the amount of food consumed, thus contributing to weight loss.

More specifically, here are some of the things we know through recent research:

- People who drink two cups of water right before eating consume 75 to 90 fewer calories during that meal.

- Drinking an increased amount of water results in weight loss in dieting women that is completely independent of physical activity and calorie restriction.

- In a study of middle-aged adults, those given 500 ml (about 16 ounces) of water 30 minutes before eating lost between four and five pounds over a three-month period. This was the only intervention and the only lifestyle change.

- In another study of young adults, those who drank 500 ml three times a day for two months lost weight—again independent of any other weight-loss intervention.

This is what we're interested in—losing unwanted pounds, achieving and maintaining an ideal body weight, and attaining a much healthier state of being.

This is a good time to take a look at how what we've been learning all ties together. Previously we considered the multiple benefits of physical activity. Exercise, especially resistance training—such as using free weights—builds muscle mass, which burns more calories, especially from fat stores, thus improving our lipid levels. Burning more calories reduces our weight, which lowers our blood pressure and improves our glucose levels.

But in the process, waste products are produced that need to be eliminated from our bodies. That's where our kidneys come in, doing what they do best—getting rid of these substances that we no longer need and that can cause damage when allowed to accumulate. That elimination takes water—enough to keep our kidneys flushing out these toxins.

That's the way God designed our bodies to work, and it all flows together, doesn't it? And it all requires an adequate amount of water.

"But how much is enough? And what if I just don't like water?"

Let's deal first with the "how much" part.

The old adage, "Make sure you drink eight glasses of water a day," probably still holds. But those need to be eight-ounce glasses. That amount correlates well with the current guidelines of about three quarts of liquid a day for men and a little less for women. I hope you noticed the word *liquid*. It doesn't all have to come from water, though that would be the easiest way of assuring an adequate intake. Other sources of liquid are other sugar-free beverages, as well as fruits and vegetables. Some of these contain a lot of water. So that helps answer the question about not liking water. Each of us can find *something* we like to drink or eat.

This is another area where keeping a journal would be very helpful, even for only a couple of days. Just record the amount of water and other beverages you consume daily, and see how it stacks up against that three-quart goal. You'll probably be surprised. You just might not be getting as much as you think. I know that unless I pay attention, I fall short and don't drink enough water.

Keep in mind that amount is intended for *routine*, everyday life. If you're planning to engage in vigorous and prolonged exercise, you'll need to increase that goal. A hot, humid environment will also increase your needs, as will becoming sick. I remind my ill patients of the need to increase their fluid intake, and I point out the vicious cycle that can quickly develop. We feel bad and don't drink enough water or other liquids. Then we become dehydrated, feel even worse, and drink even less. That's one of the times when we really need to pay attention to how much we're drinking.

For those other times, here are some tips for ensuring an adequate fluid intake and using water as a weight-loss tool:

1. Choose things to drink that you enjoy (just not with any sugar). Calorie-free flavored products are okay, but need to be limited to one a day.

2. Drink water throughout the day.

3. Drink something with every snack and especially with each meal.

4. Eat more fruits and vegetables. Remember, this is another good source of water, maybe as much as 15 to 20 percent of our daily needs.

5. Keep a bottle of water in your car or at your desk at work.

6. While increasing your water intake, cut down on your salt. This will help you lose excess water weight.

"But how will I know if I'm getting enough water each day?"

Even if you don't keep a log, you can count on your kidneys to provide this answer. If your urine is pale yellow and odorless, you're doing fine. If it's dark yellow and you notice a strong smell, you need to be drinking more. Keep in mind that our first morning urine is normally concentrated, so don't judge things by that.

"Is it possible to drink too much water?"

A medical school pathology instructor once told us that anything can be a poison.

A fellow classmate who was awake and paying attention asked, "What about oxygen?"

"High concentrations of oxygen can cause permanent lung damage to newborn babies being cared for in a neonatal unit."

"Well, what about water?" the student persisted.

"Water intoxication is a well-defined entity, with the patient ingesting copious amounts of water, resulting in significant electrolyte derangements. Fortunately, it occurs only in patients with a psychiatric disorder, and only very rarely."

I can speak to the "very rarely" part. In almost 40 years of practicing medicine, I've never had a patient get in trouble with drinking too much water. (I probably shouldn't have said that. After all, anything is possible.)

The bottom line here is, adequate water intake is very important to our good health, and it is frequently overlooked. And now we know it's an important part of any weight-loss effort. Make sure you're drinking enough.

Cheers!

19

What Am I Supposed to Be Eating?

I wish there were an easy answer to this question. It would make things a lot simpler for my patients and for me. The reality is there is no one single answer, no supreme guideline that works for everyone. Each of us is different with unique metabolisms, assorted health conditions, and maybe most importantly, distinctive tastes and preferences. Oh, and we each come with our own set of weaknesses, especially concerning what we put into our stomachs.

However, there *is* good news here. We continue to learn more about how our bodies handle the three major food groups—proteins, fats, and carbohydrates. And we continue to learn how what we eat can either improve our health or have a negative impact. We now know some acquired diseases are connected to what and how much we eat.

Because of this ongoing research and expanding knowledge, we are able to make recommendations regarding specific diets and dietary trends. Later we'll look at some of these, but for now, there seems to be significant agreement with the following guidelines:

- Limit total fat to 30 percent of your daily caloric intake.
- Avoid trans fats like the plague.
- Olive oil is preferable to every other cooking oil.
- Daily cholesterol intake should be less than 300 mgs.

- Avoid sugar (also like the plague), including sugar-sweetened beverages.
- Increase daily water intake (six to eight eight-ounce glasses).
- Limit naturally sweetened juice (no added sugar) to four to six ounces a day (yes, that means orange juice).
- Increase daily fiber intake to at least 15 grams.
- Limit salt intake.
- Limit or avoid processed foods.
- Limit carbohydrate intake as much as possible.
- Include lean meats and fish while reducing animal fat.

Most of these just make common sense, and while there are a lot of "limits" in that list, those are things we need to watch closely. We'll talk about why these are important a little later. But for right now, these are some general guidelines to keep in mind. How each of us decides to eat and what diet we choose to follow will be a unique decision. But it's an important one, with far-reaching and significant implications. That's why we're going to spend some time considering this topic.

In the meantime, here's a sobering statement worth thinking about...

> If it comes out of a can, or a box, or a wrapper, or through a fast-food window, it eventually is going to kill you.

20

What Diet Choices Are There?

Several. But before we look at these, we need to consider some important things about what and how much we choose to eat.

First, while it sounds simple enough, we frequently either forget or misunderstand the cornerstone of weight management: The rate at which we lose weight is directly related to the difference of our energy intake and our energy needs. Breaking this down even further, in order to lose weight we must burn up more than we take in.

There's a general rule that will help us with this. Each of us has a tipping point—the amount of daily calories above which we gain weight and below which we lose it. That number turns out to be around 10 calories per pound of body weight. So if you weigh 150 pounds, your tipping point will be 1500 calories a day. And if you weigh 180 pounds, it's 1800 calories. There's some leeway with this number, and our age and gender will have an impact. But this is a reasonable estimate of what our target needs to be.

Second, while we need to be aware of the number of calories we consume each day, this can't be our only focus. Whichever diet we choose has to contain an adequate amount of the essential nutrients we need to keep our bodies functioning. Some diets—I'm talking fads here—severely limit calorie intake, which predictably results in weight loss. But by definition, these diets involve unusual food combinations or eliminations, or peculiar eating schedules. None of these should be in your list of diet choices.

Now let's consider the types of diets we can consider. Keep in mind that a major determinant of a successful weight-loss effort has to do with our adherence to a reasonable diet. And that adherence depends on our understanding and enjoyment of what we've chosen to eat. Long-term success will depend on a long-term commitment, and viewing what we eat not as a diet but as a lifestyle.

The main categories of acceptable diets are briefly described below. We'll be looking at these in more detail a little later.

Balanced, Low-Calorie Diets

This is the most basic of our choices. We simply use the currently accepted composition standard of 30 percent fat, 50 percent carbohydrates, and 20 percent protein to determine what we should be eating. Then we reduce our daily calorie intake to some achievable level—usually 1500 or less—and choose the foods we want to eat. Our problem is that the average American diet contains more fat than 30 percent, as well as more carbs and less protein, thus requiring a careful analysis of what we put on our plates. With this approach, alcohol, sugary beverages, and highly concentrated sweets will need to be eliminated. These are major sources of empty calories, and their exclusion from any serious weight-loss effort makes a lot of sense.

Portion-Controlled Diets

This is a relatively easy way to reduce our daily caloric intake to a predetermined goal. We simply utilize prepackaged meals as well as frozen food, nutrition bars, and formula diet drinks. These would be the familiar weight-loss plans such as Jenny Craig and Nutrisystem. Care needs to be taken to ensure that adequate levels of essential vitamins and minerals are being met. These programs can be effective and educational, but they're not intended for long-term use.

Low-Fat Diets

This is just what it sounds like—reducing the amount of fat in our daily diet. Most experts recommend lowering our fat intake to less than 30 percent of total calories. Since each gram of fat contains a little more than 9 calories, the 150-pound individual we considered above should limit their daily fat intake to less than 45 grams per day. This will require our reading food labels and learning the nutritional content of what we eat, but that's something we need to be doing anyway. And as a general guideline, if something "melts in your mouth," it probably has fat in it.

Low-Carbohydrate Diets

As with the low-fat diet, this approach is just what it sounds like—reduced carbohydrate intake. Once again, when we consider the same 150-pound person, keeping in mind that each gram of carbohydrate contains 4 calories, the standard dietary composition of 50 percent carbs would give us a total of almost 200 grams of carbohydrates each day. To put that amount into perspective, most proponents of the low-carb approach recommend 60 to 100 grams per day at a maximum, with less than 60 being the preferred target. A few rabid adherents say that less than 30 grams should be the goal. Whatever our reduction of carbs, we'll need to make up the calories somewhere, and that will either be with fat or protein. The successful low-carb dieters increase their protein intake, choosing lean meats, fish, and chicken. This dietary choice can become a lifestyle change and thus a long-term diet.

High-Protein Diets

We'll briefly mention this since we'll probably come across it as we study various types of diets. This is simply a remodeling of that standard nutritional composition, with a greater percentage of protein being included—as much as 35 to 40 percent rather than the accepted 20 percent. This can get tricky, since those of us with kidney disease should be monitoring our protein intake. Yet for many, choosing a diet higher in protein can result in a greater ability to maintain weight loss. As with other manipulations of nutritional components, we need to be sure we're meeting our requirements of essential vitamins and minerals. While the high-protein diet is acceptable for many of us, there are better alternatives.

So there are our choices. Now we'll take a more detailed look at these and see which one makes the most sense for you.

21

The Fad Diets

They Come and Go

"If it's too good to be true..." Well, there's your answer—it probably is. That's time-tested wisdom for most areas in our lives, and it sure is when it comes to losing weight. If there were a magic bullet out there, we'd all be skinny and the title of this book would be *60 Ways to Get Rid of Your Oversized Clothes*. But there's no bullet and no surefire way of losing weight. Yet the Internet abounds with a multitude of claims for products and gimmicks and "new discoveries" that will "burn off those unwanted pounds"— all coming with a price. Too good to be true.

The same applies to the confusing array of weight-loss diets. By now, we should have a good grasp of what a healthy and sustainable diet looks like and how we can manipulate that to help us lose weight. It takes effort, and in order to be successful, the process will be gradual.

But most of us are human, and the shortest distance between two points is...the shortcut. We look for the easy way, the quickest way, the least painful way. This defect in our emotional makeup frequently gets us into trouble, and with regard to weight loss, makes us vulnerable to falling prey to the many schemes devised to confuse and ensnare. Let's consider what this looks like with some of the fad diets that have appeared on the scene, been proven to be ineffective, and then (thankfully) just faded away. You'll be familiar with some of these, while a few others will be obscure but nonetheless of interest.

The Grapefruit Diet

This is one of the oldest fads and focuses on the inclusion of grape-fruit—either the fruit or the juice—with each meal. Because strict adher-ence to this plan severely reduces calorie intake (as few as 800 calories a day), weight loss is anticipated and is usually rapid. But this is just another form of starvation and not possible for long-term use. And it can be dan-gerous because of the elimination of essential nutrients.

The Cabbage Soup Diet

This is what you'd expect—a diet composed of cabbage soup, con-sumed three times a day. You're only advised to do this for one week, and encouraged to drink a lot of water and take a high-quality vitamin tablet along with it. There are several variations (how is that possible?), but the theme is the same. One website recommends their line of spices to break the monotony of the soup, thus helping us make it through the week. This is touted as a kick start for a more moderate eating plan, and while some advocates note the complications of "confusion and light-headedness," these allegedly will be well worth the results of the rapid weight loss. Sounds like another plan for starvation and the beginning of a yo-yo cycle.

The Pritikin Diet

You might remember this diet, which appeared around 1980. The book describing it became a bestseller, and the focus was on "natural" foods, such as black beans, pintos, fruits, whole grains, lean meat, and seafood, though the acceptable list of foods is limited. The program also recom-mended increasing physical activity to at least 30 minutes of aerobic exer-cise a day, along with resistance training and stretching. All of this sounds good, but the diet limited or eliminated important nutrients while signif-icantly reducing calorie intake—to the point of near-starvation. It's been called a fad because of predictable side effects and the difficulty with long-term adherence. It shouldn't be this hard to find a diet you can live with long-term.

The Alkaline Diet

This diet makes a lot of sense if you're a manufacturer of urine test strips. The plan involves checking your urine several times each day to be sure you're not becoming "too acidic." According to the diet program, that's bad and needs to be avoided and corrected by eating the right foods.

Things to be spurned are fish, poultry, meat, and dairy products, as well as caffeine, sugar, and processed foods.

One of the flaws with this thinking is the management of urinary acidity/alkalinity—the pH. Within a broad range, what we eat won't affect this measurement, since our bodies—especially our kidneys—are tasked with balancing the amounts of acids and bases in our system. So as a diet, this won't work, and eliminating many of these "acid-forming" foods can prove dangerous to our health. Yet if you want to test your urine a couple of times each day, this might be for you.

The Blood-Type Diet

This proves that the human mind can dream up just about anything. The premise here is that the foods we eat react with our particular blood type, either positively or negatively. Once we know our blood type, we can determine which foods we need to eat and which to avoid. For example, those of us who are type A should be vegetarians, while those who are type O should eat lean meats, fruits and vegetables, and avoid wheat and dairy. If we happen to be type B, we'll need to stay away from corn, chicken, tomatoes, peanuts, and wheat. If you think this is nonsense, you're correct. There's no science backing up any of this, yet it has its adherents. Just goes to show…

There are other interesting ideas out there, including the baby-food diet and the various cookie diets (the Hollywood Cookie Diet and the Smart for Life Cookie Diet). You can draw your own conclusions about these. Just keep in mind that any diet that limits calorie intake to 500 to 1000 a day will result in weight loss. The question has to always be, is it healthy? If it doesn't make any sense or sounds too good to be true, you're on the way to finding that answer.

Lastly, from a theological viewpoint, there's an interesting diet that does not fall into the fad category, but in reality makes a lot of sense. This is the Daniel Fast (which is not the same as the Daniel Plan), and it's based on the Old Testament book of Daniel. This involves a 21-day avoidance of foods declared to be "unclean" in the Law of Moses, found in the Pentateuch. As an example, many types of meat were precluded, as were sweets.

In the story of Daniel, he and some of his friends only ate food derived from plants. Today, that would include fruits, whole grains, vegetables, olive oil, and seeds, while excluding processed foods, caffeine, alcohol, additives, and preservatives. As we read this account, we'll appreciate that this was one of the first RCTs (randomly controlled trials) ever recorded. Daniel and his group were the study group, while those in the palace (who continued to eat "royal foods") were the other. By the end of the study period, Daniel and his friends were much healthier than the others (Daniel 1:8-20). Not only did they appear healthier, but "in every matter of wisdom and understanding about which the king questioned them, he found them ten times better than all the magicians and enchanters in his whole kingdom."

Ten times better. That's impressive, and who could argue with someone who survived the lions' den or the fiery furnace?

22

Why Low-Fat Diets Don't Work

There are a couple of cornerstones when it comes to managing our weight, and our diet—what we choose to put into our bodies—is arguably the most important. Sadly, it's also the most difficult to get our hands around. (Getting our hands around a double cheeseburger is much easier.) But we haven't had a lot of guidance in this regard. In fact, somebody's got some 'splainin' to do.

In the early 1980s, the medical community was beginning to piece together the connection between elevated cholesterol levels and the risk of developing heart disease. The incidence of cardiovascular disease was rapidly rising, hand in hand with the obesity epidemic. Something needed to be done. Cholesterol—and by association red meats, bacon, fatty foods (especially saturated fats)—became the whipping boy of a progressive movement to improve the health of our nation and reduce the rampant heart disease that was taking its toll in lives lost and dollars spent.

But we were wrong. It turns out the real culprit here was not cholesterol and fatty foods, but carbohydrates, and more specifically, *high glycemic carbohydrates.*

Let's take a look at the evidence. When we began to eliminate cholesterol (and fat) from our diets, we had to replace it with something. That something became carbohydrates—grains, cereal, pasta, bread, potatoes. After all, we have only three categories of nutrients from which to choose: fats, carbs, and proteins. We have largely chosen carbs—the comfort foods—and we've become addicted. Cholesterol became the persona non grata, and "cholesterol-free" became the mantra of the food industry.

Still is. I recently picked up a bag of roasted peanuts in the shell and noticed in bold print, "A cholesterol-free snack." Excuse me? Of course peanuts are cholesterol-free, as is everything else not of animal origin. Yet I did feel a little healthier as I paid for my peanuts at the checkout counter.

But let's get back to the evidence, and it's pretty sobering. We've been pushing this "fat-free" business for almost 40 years. Surely by now we would be seeing some positive results. What about the incidence of heart disease? Has it plummeted? Of course not. We may be seeing a bit of a leveling off, but this is thought to be due to a multitude of factors, including better treatments, more awareness and screening, and a gradual reduction in the rate of cigarette smoking. But we're certainly not seeing the precipitous drop that had been hoped for.

What about the obesity epidemic? After all, obesity is closely tied to the onset of premature heart disease, as well as to the development of several other major problems. We all know the answer to this question—the epidemic continues to explode, and not just in this country. Over the past 30 years, the worldwide incidence of obesity has increased by almost 30 percent in adults. Alarmingly, that number rises to almost 50 percent in our children. One out of every two. But where is this happening? We know we have a problem in the United States, but in what other parts of the world are we seeing this explosion of obesity?

The World Health Organization (WHO) has recently published data that lists the ten countries that account for more than half of the earth's obese population. In addition to the United States, those nations are India, China, Brazil, Russia, Indonesia, Mexico, Egypt, Germany, and Pakistan. Some of these might surprise you, but that's what WHO has reported.

Many factors are involved in this epidemic, including a progressive decrease in the amount of regular physical exercise we are getting and, in this country at least, the pervasiveness of fast-food restaurants. We're just not eating right. But it's not the red meat that's doing this—it's the relentless move to reduce fats in our diet, which we've replaced with more high-glycemic-index carbs. What are we talking about here?

Let's start with the *glycemic index* (GI). This is a system of comparing the relative amounts of sugar in various foods and how rapidly they release glucose into our bloodstream. The higher the index rating, the faster glucose is released, the more rapid the rise of our blood-sugar levels, and the more insulin required to get that level under control. A lower index rating still releases glucose into our system, but at a more controlled, manageable rate.

For the sake of simplicity, this index uses pure glucose as the gold standard and assigns it a value of 100. Everything else is pegged to this number. Here are some examples:

- low-GI foods (55 or less): avocadoes, beans, almonds, peanuts, whole intact grains

- medium GI foods (56 to 69): grape juice, raisins, honey, not intact whole grains, bananas

- high GI foods (70 to 100): whole wheat bread, corn flakes (92!), pretzels, bagels, potatoes

If you take a close look here, you won't see any meats or fats listed. Remember, proteins and fats don't contain any carbs, and fruits and vegetables don't contain any cholesterol. The GI of corn flakes is surprising, as is that for a baked potato (85). Table sugar comes in at 58, placing it in the medium range.

Why is this important? In a nutshell (no cholesterol here), high-glycemic foods trigger a rapid release of insulin, which as we know does a lot of bad things. It tells the body to make and store fat for that potential rainy day, which we all know is not coming. In those of us who get little exercise, this body fat is deposited around our trunk—a pattern that we now know is associated with hyperlipidemia and an increased risk of heart disease. Additionally, high-GI foods, because of rapidly rising and falling blood-sugar levels, trigger a hunger response, causing us to eat more (usually more carbs) and gain more weight.

If all of this is valid, we would be seeing an increase in obesity in this country. And guess what?

If you want to gain a deeper understanding of this problem, I recommend two books. The first is *Grain Brain* by David Perlmutter, a neurologist (Little, Brown and Company, 2013). The other is *Wheat Belly* by

William Davis, a cardiologist (Rodale Books, 2011). Be prepared—they're not for the faint of heart.

So if our current low-fat/high-carb approach is killing us (and killing our efforts to lose weight) what are we supposed to be eating? And how do we make that change?

It might not be as difficult as you think.

23

The Low-Carbohydrate Approach

We're all a little different, and one size doesn't fit all, whether it's the clothes we wear, our choice of movies, or the cars we drive. We embrace the idea of being our own person. That's certainly a factor when it comes to determining the best dietary approach for each individual. One diet doesn't fit all. But here *is* something that comes close to being a constant, and that is that every one of us needs to limit our carbohydrate intake—some more than others.

But what's so bad about carbs? Why the rap against our comfort foods? Let's start with the real culprit here—*insulin*. This is going to be a little refresher in physiology, but it's something we really need to understand, especially as to how it relates to weight gain (and hopefully loss).

We all know that our bodies need energy to grow and survive. We get that from three sources: carbohydrates, proteins, and fat. We are able to derive energy from each of these classes of nutrients, but carbs are the easiest, quickest source—and in the long run, the most harmful. That's because in order to utilize the energy in carbs, we must recruit the action of the hormone insulin.

Insulin is made in the "beta cells" of the pancreas and is a relatively simple chain of 51 amino acids. Its release is signaled by the presence of carbohydrates in our bloodstream. When this process is initiated, insulin circulates throughout the body, seeking and attaching itself to insulin receptors. These are chemical binders located on the membranes of "target cells," and once the insulin molecule combines with this receptor, the hormone is able to exert its actions, which are many.

Insulin directly or indirectly affects almost every tissue in our body. These actions are complex and interwoven, but right now, we're going to mainly consider how it interacts with glucose and how it affects the production of energy. It does this by its action on three tissues: the liver, muscles, and adipose tissue (fat).

Glucose—the simplest and most basic sugar—can be immediately used for energy throughout the body, or it can be stored in the liver as glycogen. Once stored, this complex of modified glucose molecules can be readily and rapidly used as an energy source when needed. Lastly, excess glucose can be converted into fat and stored in our adipose tissue. Getting the energy out of this fat takes a little longer and is a more complex process than burning available glucose. That's why our bodies first burn and deplete the available glucose and then our glycogen stores before finally turning to our adipose tissue. And that's one of the reasons it's so hard to get rid of unwanted fat and to lose weight.

Now let's consider how insulin impacts our metabolism of glucose. Every carbohydrate we put into our body eventually becomes glucose—some quicker than others. But even the highly touted complex carbohydrates end up as circulating glucose. All of the carbs, from simple to complex, end up as this simple sugar and all activate the release of insulin.

The first thing this hormone does is move glucose into the cells of various tissues. As we noted earlier, this is done by attaching itself to the cell's insulin receptor. You may have heard of or even been told that you have some degree of "insulin resistance." This is the location where that resistance takes place. The receptors seem to wear down over time after repeatedly being called into action (through a persistently high-carb diet). More and more insulin is required to activate the signal and allow glucose to enter the cell. You see where this leads—more and more insulin required to do the same amount of work and handle the same sugar load. The beta cells of the pancreas finally say, "I'm getting too old for this," and stop working. And that condition? Right—adult-onset diabetes. If this theory is correct, and considering our colossal consumption of carbohydrates, we should have an epidemic of diabetes on our hands. And guess what. We do.

But back to the actions of insulin. It drives glucose into the cells of the liver, where it stimulates the formation of a storage complex called glycogen. It drives glucose into the cells of muscle, where it can be immediately burned for energy. And it drives glucose into the cells of our adipose tissue, where it promotes the storage of triglycerides in our fat cells.

This is a good time to consider why insulin has been called "the hormone of plenty." When we have plenty to eat, and a lot of glucose circulating throughout our bodies, insulin rapidly converts some of this to needed energy. The rest is stored away for a rainy day—in the form of glycogen or as fat. (As most of us can attest, we have a significant capacity for storing fat, usually in places we would rather not.)

The problem with this rainy-day business is that in this country, that day never comes. Three not so square meals a day is the norm, with a few snacks thrown in for good measure. But our pancreas doesn't know that, and each time we load ourselves with carbs, insulin does what it's supposed to do: burn sugar and store fat, taking advantage of this moment of plenty and preparing for more austere, less plentiful times.

Along the way, it can elevate our blood pressures, damage the walls of our arteries, and interfere with the normal clotting that takes place in these vessels, leading to the formation of atherosclerotic plaques. And it causes us to gain weight. There is even emerging evidence that excess levels of insulin may be associated with the development of several cancers, including those of the colon, ovary, and breast.

Lest I give you a completely one-sided view of this essential hormone, insulin does some important and beneficial things. It handles glucose for us, and it is important in the growth process and in the formation of proteins. The problem is that it was never intended to handle the kinds of carbohydrate loads we throw at our pancreas.

The bottom line: We all need to reduce the amount of carbohydrates we consume. It doesn't matter whether we're talking about whole grains, complex carbs, or multigrain whatever. We need to know the carb content of what we're putting into our bodies and lower it.

That brings up a frequent and important question: What constitutes a low-carb diet? How many daily grams of carbs is okay?

Some general but useful guidelines are available here. Robert Atkins (of the Atkins Diet fame) would tell us that the cutoff should be 30 to 45 grams per day. That's hard, considering that one piece of whole-wheat bread has 23 grams, and one medium banana contains 26 grams.

A more realistic approach would be to target 60 or so grams per day, knowing that it's impossible to identify and eliminate every single carb from your diet. And we don't want to, anyway. A certain amount of carbs is essential for our well-being. We just need to find a way to limit their intake and restore the balanced diet our systems were designed to handle. It won't take something as drastic as the Atkins Diet, though that might be a good place to start for a couple of weeks. Fortunately, we have some effective alternatives, diets that will get the job done and that we can live with long-term. We'll take a look at some of these next.

(For a great discussion of our hunter-gatherer origins, I recommend the book *Protein Power* by Michael R. Eades and Mary Dan Eades. And for a complete discussion of the importance of low-carb diets, there are two books you should look at: *60 Ways to Lower Your Blood Sugar* by Dennis Pollock and *The New Sugar Busters!* by H. Leighton Steward and others. These are all great resources and will help clarify the mistakes and myths of the past few decades regarding what we should and should not be eating.)

24

The Low-Carb Diet

What It Looks Like

As we discuss some dieting options, we need to keep in mind that we're talking about lifestyle and eating-style changes. Whichever path we choose to take regarding this important part of our overall weight-loss strategy, it needs to be something we can live with over the long haul. Fads and deprivation may lead to smaller numbers on our scales, but that won't last long. The long haul—that's what our goal has to be.

Now, how does the low-carb diet fit into this long-term thinking? For me, this has become a lifestyle change. As a physician, I am convinced of the solid evidence supporting the need to limit carbohydrates in our diets. We were not designed to handle sugars and carbs very well, regardless of whether they're complex or not. From the outset, we were hunters and gatherers. It was not until we became civilized that we discovered wheat and corn and sugar. And that's when diabetes and a host of other maladies discovered us. Most experts agree that the epidemic of diabetes in this country is due to two things: physical inactivity and an ever-increasing consumption of carbohydrates. Increasing our daily exercise will yield substantial benefits, but cutting way back on our carbs dwarfs this when it comes to improving our overall health.

So how do we go about reducing our carbohydrates? There are several sources of information regarding this, but it turns out to be rather simple.

If you want a good starting point, the Atkins Diet is a reasonable place to begin. There are multiple variations of this plan, and as long as they reduce our carbohydrates to about 30 grams per day, they'll work.

Here are some sample meal plans, giving us an idea of the kinds of things we can eat while on this diet. Most of these combinations will limit our calorie intake to around 1500 per day—a good initial target.

Breakfast

- two-egg omelet with sausage, cheese, red peppers
- two poached eggs with smoked salmon and a couple slices of tomato
- 1 cup of berries, one egg (any way), ½ cup cottage cheese, 1 tablespoon of shredded cheese

Lunch

- 4 ounces of tuna fish, ½ cup of baby carrots, 2 tablespoons of hummus
- a large tossed salad with tuna or chicken and low-carb dressing
- Reuben sandwich (one slice of low-carb bread) and a green salad with low-carb dressing
- steak and pepper fajitas on a low-carb tortilla with a tossed salad

Dinner

- grilled chicken breast, steamed asparagus, and yellow squash, with a mixed salad with vinaigrette or low-carb dressing
- 5 ounces of chicken and 1 cup of broccoli, along with 8 ounces of tofu noodles and a garden salad
- roasted pork tenderloin with sautéed spinach and red peppers

Snacks

- celery sticks with low-carb dip
- olives and cheddar cheese cubes

- 1 cup of edamame
- light string cheese

There are a couple of things that need to be kept in mind. One piece of bread with one meal a day is fine, as long as it's low carb. Healthy grains, multigrains, and the like are not part of this low-carb approach. Read your labels.

It's fine to have two snacks a day—morning and afternoon. Just don't overdo it.

There is no limit to the amount of salad or veggies that you can eat with this approach. Just be sure that the chosen vegetables are on the low-carb list. For example, green beans are fine, while pinto beans, navy beans, and black-eyed peas are not. Too many carbs. And remember, low-carb salad dressings are fine while low-fat dressings are not. Too much added sugar.

This gives us an idea of what we can eat while on this diet. Once again, there are many sources of menu ideas available, and we should be able to find a plan that suits our needs and tastes.

Now let's talk turkey. Actually, that's a good protein source while on this diet. But let's consider reality, and I'm speaking from personal experience as well as that of hundreds of my patients. The low-carb approach—targeting no more than 30 grams of carbohydrates a day—will help you lose weight. But for me, it's not something I can or want to do forever. I changed my own diet to low-carb more than 15 years ago and lost around 15 pounds. And I watched my blood pressure go down as well as my cholesterol level. Surprisingly (and happily), my HDL (the *good* cholesterol) more than doubled. And while I've continued to limit my carbohydrate intake, I've gradually shifted to what I believe to be the most reasonable and healthy dietary approach. It's also something I can stick with forever—the Mediterranean Diet. We're going to look at that next.

25

What's the Best Diet?

One Clear Choice

As you can see by now, a lot of questions surround the issue of what we need to be eating. In our clinic, we are frequently asked about our dietary recommendations to help with weight loss and to help manage lipid disorders and blood-sugar problems. Again, one size doesn't fit all, and if there is a magic wand somewhere, I've yet to find it.

From a previous chapter, we've considered the failure of a low-fat diet as a healthy alternative. That leaves us with a couple of viable choices, and we'll discuss those here.

First is the Mediterranean Diet. It should be understood that there is no single definition for this diet, and in fact, the word *Mediterranean* might be somewhat of a misnomer. The name is used to refer to a way of eating that is high in fruits, vegetables, whole grains, beans, nuts (especially walnuts and almonds), and seeds. Additionally, there is low to moderate intake of fish and poultry and little red meat. Wine consumption (low to moderate amounts) is acceptable, and olive oil is a mainstay. There are numerous books on the subject, as well as dietary plans and menus. But does it make sense?

Several large and recent studies indicate the answer is yes. When compared to a low-fat diet, use of the Mediterranean Diet demonstrates a significantly reduced incidence in the rates of cardiovascular events (strokes, heart attacks, and cardiovascular deaths). Interestingly, there appears to be a reduced incidence in the development of Parkinson's disease and Alzheimer's. And significantly, this diet also appears to lower the chances of developing type 2 diabetes.

Notice that the inclusion of olive oil is foundational to this diet, and while most olive oils will be fine, I'd recommend the extra virgin varieties, and the cold pressed if you can find them. They'll cost a little more, but the difference in taste is noticeable, and some believe they have fewer impurities and more natural nutrients. Whichever type of olive oil you decide to use, it should become the mainstay of your cooking oils.

Now the South Beach Diet. This was developed by a cardiologist and dietician, and was done so as an alternative to the low-fat diet. The diet has become very popular, and you can find a lot of books and plans on its use. What sets it apart from other diets is the focus on good carbs versus bad carbs.

The good carbs are those with a lower glycemic index: most vegetables, beans, and whole grains. And the bad carbs are on the other end of the glycemic index spectrum: processed grains, sugars, potatoes.

As you can see, this diet is not really focused on being low-carb, and I'm not sure the body can differentiate very well between a good carb and a bad one. Mounting medical evidence would agree. Yet the South Beach Diet does move us away from the exclusion of meat and fat. That's a good thing, since we know that strategy just doesn't work.

Lastly, we need to address the DASH diet. I'm asked about this from time to time in our office, and I explain to my patients that this is not really a weight-loss diet or a means of lowering your cholesterol. The acronym stands for Dietary Approach to Stop Hypertension, and it's effective in doing that. It stresses the inclusion of fruits and vegetables while limiting the amount of low-fat dairy products and lean meats. It's also rich in potassium, magnesium, and calcium—minerals that are efficient in lowering blood pressure. And as we noted, strict adherence to this diet is an effective weapon in the battle to control blood pressure, and it may also help us lose some weight.

So where does that leave us? Is there one specific diet we should try? One diet that stands out from the rest? The answer is yes, and the winner is…the Mediterranean Diet.

I advise my patients to familiarize themselves with the key elements of this diet and make some minor alterations to it. This includes more lean meats and less grains. Nuts are great for snacking, especially walnuts and almonds. And as already mentioned, olive oil (the extra virgin variety if you can afford it) should occupy a prominent place in your pantry. This diet is really a lifestyle change and requires understanding and commitment. Not that it's hard to do—quite the contrary. It's just that it's unlike what we Americans are accustomed to eating. That's beginning to change, and this has the potential to make a big difference in the health of our population.

Before we move on from the importance of what we eat to help us lose weight and maintain that loss, one important point needs to be made. If your healthcare provider advises you to stick to a low fat–low cholesterol diet to help you lose weight, or for any health reason, it's time to find a new provider. It won't work, and may very well make matters worse, such as your lipid levels. Remind him or her that several large head-to-head studies comparing low-fat to low-carb diets clearly give the thumbs-up to low carbohydrates. Fewer deaths, less heart disease, less diabetes, and more and sustainable weight loss. They should know better.

Hot off the Press!

A recent article in a trustworthy and respected medical journal just reported a study comparing the Mediterranean Diet with a low-fat diet. What they found was fascinating and potentially a game-changer. Those people who consumed the Mediterranean Diet—with either additional nuts or additional olive oil—had less cognitive impairment (dementia) than those on a low-fat diet. In fact, those who increased their weekly olive oil intake to one liter (a little more than four cups) demonstrated an improvement in their cognitive abilities. This is a preliminary study and further work will either support or refute these findings, but if valid, this could have significant implications. Four cups may be a lot of olive oil in a week, and the actual amount that confers this benefit might be less. We'll need to wait and see. But here's some advice worth remembering...

Let food be thy medicine and medicine be thy food.

Hippocrates

26

The Mediterranean Diet

What It Looks Like

As I said a few pages back, the Mediterranean Diet is the place where most of us need to be. No, probably all of us. We'll see many variations on this theme, but the components of this diet are straightforward. We looked at these in the last chapter, and it's important to keep the following in mind:

- Extra virgin olive oil (preferred) and canola oil should be used instead of butter (though a small amount is okay).
- Fresh fruit and vegetables are a major part of this diet and include tomatoes, spinach, eggplant, cucumbers, and bell peppers.
- The main sources of protein include fish, chicken, and beans.
- Nuts, eggs, and seeds are other acceptable sources of protein.
- Parmesan and other savory cheeses, as well as Greek yogurt, are good sources of calcium while adding flavor to our meals.

Here are some menu ideas this diet has to offer:

Breakfast
- 6 ounces of Greek yogurt topped with ½ cup of raspberries/ blueberries/strawberries and 1 teaspoon of honey

- granola and milk plus an omelet of your choice

Lunch
- grape leaves stuffed with walnut salad
- roast beef and feta salad
- turkey/chicken salad with slices of tomato and a cup of minestrone soup

Dinner
- chicken kabobs with basmati rice and vegetables of your choice
- 3 ounces of salmon, asparagus spears, and a green salad

Snacks
- fresh fruit
- almonds
- roasted soybeans

Dessert
- small bunch of grapes
- ½ cup of lemon sorbet

While not an exhaustive list of the things we should eat, it does give us an idea of what this diet can look like. And it really shouldn't be viewed as a diet but as a lifestyle way of eating. As a weight-loss tool, it can easily be adapted for success by limiting our calorie intake to 1500 per day.

As we noted at the outset, the Mediterranean Diet makes the most sense for most of us. A simple and quick Google search will overwhelm us with menu ideas, and each of us will be able to find a wide variety of items and dishes to choose from. My advice here is to keep it simple, and don't complicate your life any more than it has to be. Weight loss and maintenance doesn't have to be a chore. That's right. It can be tasty and even fun.

27

"He Created Them Male and Female"

This chapter is dedicated to my wife, Barbara. For years she has maintained that women lose weight differently than men, and that what works for men might not do so for the fairer sex. I hope she doesn't read this because it turns out she was right. This is complex physiology, and we are just now beginning to unravel some of the mystery, but there are several things we know. And we're beginning to understand how the differences between men and women determine much about how we gain and lose weight.

Let's start with what's considered to be normal body composition. For a woman, that would be a body fat between 20 and 30 percent. For a man, the range is less—12 to 20 percent. Men have more lean muscle mass and tend to burn more energy and calories while at rest. It also seems that men burn more calories while exercising, making it easier for men to eat more without gaining weight and to lose weight faster than women.

We also know that women store fat quicker than men, but in turn burn it in preference to other energy sources while exercising. The reasons for this variation are unknown, but may relate to the different actions of testosterone and estrogen, differences in the way the two sexes handle glucose, and the higher levels of leptin in women. Leptin is a hormone that inhibits hunger, and we'll be taking a good look at this later.

In addition to the differences in the way men and women handle fat, women while at rest burn more glucose (from carbohydrate sources) than do men. And stress affects women differently as well, causing the inhibition of fat loss.

As we noted, all of this is complex and still being sorted out. So how do we put what we currently know to good use? First, since women preferentially turn to fat as a fuel during exercise, it becomes really important to take advantage of this by encouraging moderate physical activity with any weight-loss effort. Some research indicates that resistance exercise (weight training) stimulates the release of body fat from fat cells, causing it be quickly burned as fuel. If that's the case—and it seems to be—then we should be recommending the inclusion of resistance training to our daily exercise routine. It doesn't have to be every day, but a couple of times each week.

This is a good place to debunk the idea that women lose less weight than men with the same amount of exercise. This has been the prevailing view for a long time, and you might have heard or read about this inequality. A recent and comprehensive study looked at this and the conclusions are clear. While there are differences in fuel sources and calories burned, there is no evidence for sex differences in body weight response to exercise. We all need to be moving, and probably pumping a little iron while we're at it.

Finally, since women store fat faster than men, the dietary choices for women should focus on less fat intake. This can still work with the low-carb or Mediterranean diets, but we'll need to pay attention to the sources and amounts of fat in our meals.

So yes, Barbara, there is a difference between males and females when it comes to losing weight. You've been right all along.

28

Getting It Wrong

Cindy Stewart

"Strange case in room 5."

John Tucker, one of my partners, tossed a chart onto the countertop of the ER nurses' station and scratched the top of his head.

"Oh yeah? What's going on?" I finished the record of the patient in the ortho room and dropped it into the discharge basket.

"Twenty-year-old woman with blurred vision and some dizziness. Everything checks out okay. Blood pressure is fine, no neurological problems, and her heart sounds fine. Her vision testing is completely normal, so I can't explain the visual changes."

"What about her blood sugar?" (The elevated blood sugar of new-onset diabetes can cause the tension in your eyeball to change, blurring your vision—always something to think about.)

"Completely normal. And all the rest of her blood work is fine too. I think I'll get an MRI just to be sure everything's all right in her brain."

So far this didn't sound very strange. We see a lot of people with dizziness and vague complaints, and usually they pan out to be nothing serious. I glanced at Cindy Stewart's chart in front of John.

"What's so strange about Ms. Stewart, John?"

He was still scratching his head and squinting his eyes. "Just something about the way she's acting. It's not all coming together. She's a student at USC and doing really well—prelaw, she tells me. And she's always been healthy and active. Runs every day. Plays racquetball. But there's just something…I don't know. Maybe I'm overreacting. I'll get that MRI and if it's normal, I'll send her home and let her follow up with her family doctor."

I nodded and picked up the chart of the next patient to be seen. Before I headed to their room, something stopped me. I learned long ago to always trust my gut. I was about to remind John of that, but he was gone, heading down the hallway.

John sent Cindy home that day, shortly after the MRI of her head came back completely normal. Her dizziness had improved a little, and he told her to follow up with her family doctor.

That didn't happen, and three weeks later she showed back up in the ER. This time it was three in the morning, and EMS 3 was rolling her into the cardiac room.

"Tell me what's going on," I said to Denton Roberts, the lead paramedic.

He and his partner were carefully transferring the young woman from their stretcher to ours. That's when I noticed Cindy's flushed face. I placed the back of my hand against her cheek. She was burning.

"We got the call from her friend's house," Denton began, catching his breath and wiping sweat from his forehead. "Unresponsive and a high fever was what we were told. Her blood pressure's low—70 over 40—and she's got some kind of rash on her back and legs. I'm wondering if she has meningitis or something like that."

Lori Davidson was starting an IV in Cindy's left arm. "I'll get a temp in a second, but she's on fire. Must be 103 or more."

I glanced at her legs, looking for the rash Denton reported. On the back of both calves were more than two dozen angry, ulcerated lesions. Not the typical rash we see with meningococcal meningitis. Yet it was something to consider, and we had to be careful.

"Any of her friends come with her?"

Denton looked at me and shook his head. "Sorta typical. We got to the house, they told us she was sick, and when we turned around, they were gone. That's all the info we got. Don't know anything about her medical history or any prescription medications."

We *did* know about her dizziness and visual changes from her previous visit, but John hadn't mentioned any significant medical history or prescription medications. Amy Connors, our unit secretary, would be pulling Cindy's old record so we would be able to check on any available history.

"Temp's 106!" Lori exclaimed. "I'll get the cooling blanket. Anything else we need right now?"

"Get the lab down here," I answered, putting my hand on Cindy's forehead. If possible, she was even hotter than before. I leaned close and called her name. No response. "We'll need the usual blood studies and a couple sets of blood cultures. When you get the chance, start another IV and let's chill those fluids. We need to cool her down."

A flurry of activity exploded in the room—organized chaos. This young woman was in serious trouble.

The thought of meningitis crossed my mind again, and I lifted her head, checking for any cervical rigidity—a sign of meningeal irritation. Her neck was completely supple, and there was no reflexive drawing up of her knees. There was still no reflexive movement at all.

I took the ophthalmoscope from its holder on the wall and focused the bright light first on her left pupil, then the right. They were normal-sized and reactive—both good signs. I was moving away when something caught my attention—something barely visible, maybe just imagined. It had been a faint reflection from her right eye. I leaned closer, shining the light of the scope at an angle this time. There it was—an opacity in the middle of her eye—faint, but definite. It was a cataract.

I stepped back and took a deep breath. Why would this young woman have a cataract? And one that was so well-formed and already dense.

A quick re-exam of her left eye showed the same thing—another cataract. That would explain the blurred vision she had complained about to John Tucker. I couldn't blame John for missing these though. Cataracts are usually not considered emergencies and not something we routinely check for in the ER. They can be subtle, and I had almost missed them myself.

"What's the matter?" Lori was standing beside me, regulating the flow of chilled IV fluids flowing into Cindy's right arm.

"This just isn't adding up yet," I answered. "She has bilateral cataracts, and unless they're congenital or some sort of genetic trait, I don't know why she has them. That and the fever and rash."

The cardiac monitor beeped its alarm and both of us glanced at the monitor screen. Cindy's heart rate was now 140 and she was having

PVCs—extra beats, usually due to irritability of the heart muscle. Maybe her fever or some infection.

"107!" One of the techs called out.

Ice bags? Stomach lavage with cold water? I had never needed to do that, but we had to get her temperature down.

The door opened, and Amy Connors stepped into the room.

"Got some lab reports, Amy?" I was hoping for help from any quarter. Maybe there was an answer in those lab studies.

"No, but I have this." She stepped toward me, her outstretched hand holding a bottle of some kind. "One of this woman's friends came through the ambulance entrance and almost threw this at me. Then she took off and was gone."

She dropped what appeared to be a pill bottle into my hand. I turned it over until the label came into view.

A red, white, and blue flag was prominently displayed—the Union Jack. This was some sort of British medication, or at least that's what the manufacturer would have you believe. I scanned the label and read, "DNP. 2,4-Dinitrophenol (200mg)."

DNP. My brain flashed through the archives of my organic chemistry days. Nothing. But something more recent—something I had come across a few months earlier made its way to the front of my mind.

"This stuff is used for weight loss. Or at least it was. Illegal now because of its toxicity."

Lori looked over my shoulder at the bottle. "Maybe not illegal in England, if that's where she got it. What about its toxicity? Is there some kind of antidote or something we can do?"

It was all coming back now. I remembered thinking that the information was interesting, but it was something I had never seen and probably never would. Yet here was Cindy Stewart, experiencing all of the complications of using this deadly substance as a weight-loss supplement.

"Just supportive care is all I know to do. There's no specific antidote. We just need to get her temperature down and her blood pressure up. This explains the cataracts and rash. And her fever. This stuff causes your metabolism to shift into the highest gear possible for the human body, and you burn up calories. And burn up your insides. And your brain. If we can't get her cooled off—"

"She's seizing!"

Right before sunrise, just as Cindy Stewart's body was being wheeled down the hallway to the morgue, I had a chance to sit down in front of our computer and search the Internet for DNP. A couple of clicks and I found a picture of Cindy's pill bottle.

Fat Burner

DNP has various applications and has gained steady popularity as a fat loss aid. Boasting an astounding 50 percent increase in metabolic rate, it is able to contribute to reported fat losses of 10-12 pounds in 8 days of use. However, (for legal reasons) we do not sell this product for human consumption. We leave it up to you to decide what to do with it.

29

Complementary and Alternative Medicine (CAM)

"Doc, my nephew—whose girlfriend is in nursing school—says that if you drink three ounces of vinegar a day and stand flat against a wall for 15 minutes after eating, you can lose weight. About five pounds a week. What do you think?"

He seemed to be serious, so I needed to suppress my smile and give him a serious answer.

We're frequently asked about alternative treatments for many common ailments—with weight loss being chief among them. We want to know about their effectiveness and safety. It all depends, but first let's define these terms.

Alternative medicine refers to the use of a nonmainstream approach *in place of* conventional, mainstream medicine. *Complementary medicine* refers to using a nonmainstream approach *along with* mainstream medicine.

A true alternative approach to a medical problem—for instance, treating bacterial pneumonia with poultices—is not very common. It's much more likely we'll combine nonmainstream and conventional treatments if we're convinced of the effectiveness of both.

For our discussion here, we'll use the acronym CAM, which stands for "complementary and alternative medicine." It encompasses all the various nonmainstream treatments available to us. The margins begin to blur a little with the passage of time. What was earlier considered to be CAM has become more conventional. A few examples are the utilization of fish oil in the treatment of elevated triglyceride levels and niacin to elevate low HDL levels. Prior to that would be the native Peruvians' discovery of the medicinal use of the bark of the cinchona tree. It found widespread use as a treatment for malaria (quinine) and a cardiac medicine (quinidine), variations of which are still in use today.

How common is the use of CAM therapies in the United States? It appears that more than one in five of us will employ some form of this treatment, with the choices including acupuncture, ayurveda (a system of Hindu traditional medicine), homeopathy, Chinese or Oriental medicine, chiropractic, massage, body movement therapies, tai chi, yoga, dietary supplements, herbal medicine, biofeedback, electromagnetic therapy, qigong (balancing your chi or "life energy"), meditation, hypnosis, and even art, dance, and music. Whew.

In the US, the most frequently used CAM therapies (in descending order) are herbal remedies, breathing meditation, other forms of meditation, chiropractic manipulation, yoga, diet-based therapy, progressive relaxation, and megavitamin therapy. Interestingly, the British National Health Service lists their three most commonly employed CAM therapies as acupuncture, aromatherapy, and chiropractic. You could find some interesting combinations there.

The problem we face with CAM therapies is determining their effectiveness and safety. We have the same dilemma with our conventional treatments, whether they be pharmaceutical, surgical, or other (such as radiation therapy). It all comes down to performing rigorous and reproducible research. That takes money, and frequently a lot of it. Our pharmaceutical companies have it to spend, and they fund much (many think *too* much) of our ongoing medical research. They need to prove their latest medicines will work and are safe so they can get them to the market.

As you can imagine, there's probably not a lot of research going on with ayurveda or the use of dance for depression. When it does happen, most studies fail to demonstrate any beneficial outcomes with many CAM therapies. There have been a couple of noteworthy exceptions. The practice of tai chi has been shown to significantly reduce the incidence of falls among our elderly, probably due to better conditioning and balance. And several types of acupuncture have proven effective for selected conditions, including low-back pain and migraine headaches. Probably not better than conventional treatments and usually more expensive, but it seems to work. With the passage of time, many of these CAM therapies, or elements of them, may merge into the conventional.

Until then, I'm going to keep an open mind but rely on reputable journal reports and the results of well-designed and large studies. If you're considering a CAM therapy, talk with your physician. If she tries to discourage you and you forge ahead anyway, just be sure to let her know. After all, that next tree you chew on may be the secret to everlasting youth, or at least a cure for baldness.

And no, three ounces of vinegar a day and standing against a wall after eating aren't going to help you lose weight. Might help your posture though, but not so much your breath.

However, there are some CAM therapies that might be useful in our battle to lose weight, and we'll take a look at some of those.

30

CAM and Weight Loss

Dietary Supplements and What to Do with Them

It's that never-ending search for the magic bullet. We are bombarded with ads and claims for guaranteed weight loss if only we take a particular pill or liquid or supplement. And we're paying attention. More than two billion dollars a year worth of attention. At this moment, more than 10 percent of American adults are taking some form of a weight-loss supplement—with twice as many women as men admitting to this use. But is it helping or is it hurting? Let's see what we know.

Manufacturers of these supplements make all sorts of claims, from the ability of their products to suppress appetite, increase metabolism, reduce body fat, and of course to induce weight loss. But there is precious little evidence to support their claims. The reason for this is that the Food and Drug Administration (FDA) does not classify dietary supplements as drugs and does not require any premarket review or approval. Instead, manufacturers are responsible for determining whether or not their products are safe. Nothing about effectiveness.

And while the FDA does not allow these supplements to contain any pharmaceutical ingredients, several recent studies have demonstrated trace amounts of amphetamine-like substances in some products. Making this more difficult to detect is that the average product contains more than 10 different ingredients, with some having more than 90. Still, there is little oversight of this growing industry, and that should be concerning. And if you regularly take one or more of these supplements, what should you know and what should you do?

The answer to this can be found in two additional questions: Does the supplement you take help? And have you noticed any side effects? If the answers are no and yes, it's time to stop. But if you're not sure and want to continue taking them, or are considering some others, do some reading (other than the ads) and make an informed decision.

Here's a good place to start. We'll take a brief look at some of the more commonly used supplements and see what evidence and experience we have with them. Unfortunately, only in the past few years have extensive and well-designed clinical trials looked at some of these supplements, but more are on the way. And if the FDA gets more involved with quality, safety, and efficacy issues, all of this will become easier to figure out. For now, here's what we know.

Bitter orange. This is supposed to increase our metabolism and burn fat. There's no evidence this happens, and side effects include anxiety, chest pain, and increased blood pressure.

Calcium. We're frequently asked about this, especially about its ability to burn fat and decrease fat absorption. To date, there is no evidence supporting these claims. Side effects can occur when more than 2000 mgs are ingested each day, and can include constipation and kidney stones.

Chromium. This supplement has long been promoted as a muscle builder. It's supposed to increase muscle mass and reduce body fat. Only minimal positive effects have been observed, and these have not been consistent. Side effects can include dizziness, weakness, headache, and hives.

Ephedra. We should all know about this one and its dangerous side effects. Stay away. Nuff said.

Garcinia cambogia. This is a popular supplement now and is touted as an appetite suppressant and an inhibitor of fat formation. Again, there are no quality studies that support these claims. Headache, nausea, and GI symptoms can occur.

Green coffee bean extract. The claim is for weight loss due to less fat accumulation, and there seems to be some evidence to support this. These findings are modest, but side effects are minimal and include headache and possibly urinary symptoms. This might be a supplement to consider trying.

Green tea. This stuff (either the extract found in capsules or the beverage itself) is supposed to increase energy expenditure and reduce fat absorption. It's been around for a while, and I've followed any studies concerning its benefits, since I take the capsules myself. At this time, there is some evidence that it might have a small effect on body weight and good evidence that it's safe. I'll keep taking it.

These are just a few of the dozens, maybe hundreds, of herbal products and supplements currently being sold as weight-loss enhancers. Just be aware that none of these are FDA approved or even FDA evaluated and inspected. Know what you're taking, and be aware of the only absolute truth with any of these: There is no magic bullet.

If you didn't see your favorite supplement here and want more information, here's a great website from the National Institutes of Health: https://ods.od.nih.gov/factsheets/WeightLoss-HealthProfessional.

Three months and I've lost six pounds. Slow and steady, and no pain. Keeping that diary helped me identify some stuff I shouldn't have been eating and it educated me about reducing my portion sizes. Especially when it came to nuts. "A small handful" is the recommended amount—about a quarter cup. My handful turned out to be more than two-thirds of a cup and a lot more calories. Ya gotta measure stuff. And while six pounds may not sound like much, it's made a big difference in my waist size. Anyway, four more weeks and I'll be at my goal.

31

Okay, Doc, I Think It's Time for a Pill

Dave Jernigan was in the office for his three-month checkup, or weigh-in, as he liked to call it. He had missed his appointment last week because of a business trip to the West Coast and had insisted we work him in this morning.

"Okay, Dave, how are things going?" I closed the door and sat down beside the exam room table.

I already knew how his weight was going—he'd gained four pounds since his last visit. That might explain his fidgeting and insistence on being seen today.

"Things are not goin' so good, Doc. It must be the travel I've had to do lately and not being able to exercise or eat right. You see my chart—I'm gaining weight instead of losing it. It's time we do something different."

I glanced at Dave's record. His blood pressure continued to be fine, and his other vital signs were normal.

"Tell me how you did with the low-carb diet and your exercise plan. I thought you were on the right track there."

"I was." He shook his head and stared at the floor. "The low-carb thing is easy for me to do, except when I'm on the road. It gets pretty tough to find a decent salad at an airport or late at night in a hotel. My exercising was going great too, and I was starting to lose some weight. Then it just stopped, and I started to put the pounds back on."

This wasn't going to be the normal plateau effect that happens with weight loss. Dave was struggling with what he was eating and probably how much he was eating.

"I've done a little research, Doc. I looked into that over-the-counter stuff—orlistat—the medicine that's supposed to cut down on the absorption of fat that you eat. But I talked with a couple of guys at work that had tried it, and I don't want any of those side effects. Cramps, gas…not for me."

"Dave, you can—"

"I don't think that stuff's for me. I read about phentermine as a possibility, and I think I'd like to try that. It's an appetite-suppressant, right? That might be just what I need. And since my blood pressure has been under control for a long time, it should be safe. What do you think?"

I knew Dave pretty well, and from the tone of his voice and the look in his eye, I could tell I would be wasting my time and his trying to convince him that orlistat would be a good choice and how most of those side effects can be overcome. But phentermine was a good second option.

"Okay. But there are some things you'll need to understand about taking this medication."

We discussed how the drug worked, the side effects to watch out for, what kind of weight loss we could expect, and that he would need to closely monitor his blood pressure.

"We'll start with a one-month supply and see how things go. Remember, Dave, three months max. No more than that. In fact, if you're not losing weight after two months, we might pull the plug then."

"And the low-carb diet? I keep doing that, right?"

"Yes, and your exercise. You'll need to continue doing all those things. We're going to look at the phentermine as sort of a jump start. It will help you lose some weight, but you'll still need to manage your lifestyle—while you're on the medicine and for the rest of your life."

Dave jumped down from the exam table. "Thanks, Doc. This is gonna work. One month, right? I'll see you then."

32

Prescription Weight-Loss Medicines

Is One Right for Me?

Losing weight isn't easy. If you've ever tried it, then you know that's true. In fact, I assume that's why you picked up this book—to get some help.

Let's start once more with the basics. Every successful weight-loss effort begins with setting a goal. We've mentioned a 5 percent loss of initial body weight as not only being reasonable but worthwhile. This appears to be the point at which a lot of good things start to happen. Cardiovascular risk factors improve, the incidence of diabetes goes down, insulin sensitivity gets better (it takes less of this hormone to do the same amount of work—a good thing), and all the problems associated with excess weight begin to correct themselves.

Once we've established our goal, we decide on an appropriate change of diet, increase our exercise, and find constructive ways to modify our behavior. This last part can be as involved as seeking professional help and counseling or as simple as keeping a food diary and evaluating what we're eating. For many people, these changes may be enough to allow them to achieve their weight-loss target. For a lot of us, it won't be enough. We'll need some help.

Fortunately, help *is* available in the form of effective and safe medications. The addition of these to an overall program can produce as much as 5 to 10 percent additional weight loss. That's a lot, and it's going to bring about a lot of good changes.

But weight-loss drugs are not for everyone and shouldn't be the first thing we reach for to cast off unwanted pounds. As a physician, I have some guidance here when it comes to prescribing these medications.

Anti-obesity drugs can be added to a weight-loss program in an individual with a BMI greater than 30 who has failed to achieve their weight-loss goal through diet and exercise. The time frame here is generally around six months of sustained effort. The BMI threshold is lower (27 to 29.9) if that same individual has a *comorbid condition* such as diabetes, heart disease, elevated cholesterol, high blood pressure, sleep apnea, and significant joint disease. Some experts might begin medication from the outset if a person's BMI is greater than 35 and the need for weight loss is urgent.

So that's when it's reasonable to start a weight-loss drug. But how will we know if it's successful? Sounds like a simple question. Shouldn't we know the answer if we're losing weight? It will depend on a couple of things.

Successful weight loss with anti-obesity drugs should result in a loss of about one pound a week, fall below the 5 percent goal between three and six months, and stay at that level. If these things happen, the medication has been successful, and in many cases and with some drugs, they can be continued. But if it's not working, it's obviously time to consider a different strategy—either changing medications or focusing once again on lifestyle changes. While these drugs are largely safe, there are side effects with any medication we take, and the risk/benefit ratio has to constantly be evaluated.

That brings up a frequently asked question: How long can these diet medications safely be taken? That varies according to the type of drug, with some being safely used for more than four years. Others are intended for a much shorter period of time, measured in months—certainly less than a year. We're going to consider these differences in the next few chapters. But for now, it's important to remember that these medications are a temporary weapon in our battle with obesity, unlike diet and exercise changes, which are intended to last a lifetime.

And it's important to know that drug therapy does not *cure* obesity. Again, it's a temporary measure. When a medication has reached its maximum level of effectiveness, weight loss will stop and our weight will stabilize. That's the time to stop the medicine. We must anticipate that without significant lifestyle changes, our weight will be expected to rise. That's the challenge, but it's far from insurmountable.

Now let's consider the different types of weight-loss medications. And should you need one, we'll see which makes the most sense for you.

33

Prescription Weight-Loss Medicines, Part 1

Drugs That Alter Fat Digestion

There are three main classes of weight-loss medicines and several combinations. Let's start with one of the more common types, and certainly the safest.

It seems intuitive that if we can reduce the amount of fat that's absorbed from our GI tracts, we should be able to lose some weight. That turns out to be the case.

One drug in this class is called orlistat—you might recognize it by its trade name, Xenical. Many experts recommend orlistat for the initial treatment in those patients who need drug therapy. There are several reasons for this. The first is that it works. Since this drug has been around for a while, it has been well-studied and we know a lot about it. Of those taking this medicine, as many as 70 percent will be able to reach that "meaningful weight-loss goal" of 5 percent of their initial weight. That's a good number, though not everyone will achieve it.

In addition to being effective in helping us lose weight, orlistat does some other important things. It can reduce levels of total cholesterol and LDL, the bad cholesterol. Orlistat has also been proven to lower both systolic and diastolic blood pressures, fasting blood sugars, and to significantly reduce the risk of developing type 2 diabetes. Many of these are related to the weight loss that takes place, but some are attributed to the direct action of the drug itself.

So how does it work? It's really pretty simple. When we consume fat with our meals (remember, the average American diet contains more than 40 percent fat), several things start to happen. Chemicals are released that signal our pancreas that there's fat heading its way, and this vital digestive organ releases enzymes (lipases) that will break down these fats, thus allowing for rapid and almost complete absorption of them. Orlistat inhibits these pancreatic lipases, thus reducing the amount of fat that is broken down and absorbed. More of it is excreted through our GI tract.

This is a pretty smart drug in that in most people who eat a diet that contains around 30 percent fat, orlistat prevents about a third of this from being digested and absorbed. That appears to be the peak of its action. This is important when it comes to side effects, since as noted above, most American diets are well above that 30 percent mark.

And those side effects, while not dangerous, can be disturbing. It all has to do with the increased excretion of fat. This can result in abdominal cramps, bloating, gas, oily stools, and fecal spotting. None of that sounds very good. In fact, that's the main problem this drug had when it was first released. Again, it's effective, safe...but oily stools? The numbers tell us that less than 10 percent of people are still using orlistat after one year, and less than 1 percent after two years. Yet it's safe for longer-term use than that and will help us lose weight and keep it off. So how do we make this drug work for us? How do we reduce these side effects? And where does orlistat fit into our weight-loss program?

I tell my patients (and they quickly learn on their own) that the first step to reduce these troubling side effects is to reduce the fat in their diets. If we can get our dietary percentage of fat below 30 percent, two things happen. First, the side effects of orlistat dissipate (they tend to do this over time, anyway). And second, the reduction of fat in our diet—in and of itself—will help us lose weight. So the side effects of this medication can actually work for us. (It's hard to convince some people of that after multiple trips to the laundromat.)

Another way to reduce the incidence of these side effects is to increase the amount of fiber in our diet. This needs to be the insoluble kind—that which can't be absorbed. This type of fiber is found in whole grains, most types of beans, popcorn, broccoli, asparagus, carrots, and other vegetables and fruits. Again, increasing our fiber—just like reducing our ingestion of fat—brings with it some significant benefits.

As far as any other bothersome side effects, this drug is relatively risk-free. Very little of it is absorbed, though it can bind calcium in the gut and lead to an increased incidence of kidney stones. If you've had oxalate stones, you'll need to avoid this drug.

Now let's talk about dosing. There are prescription-strength capsules—120 mgs each—and the standard recommendation is one capsule three times a day within one hour of a meal. That's the maximum dose and will produce the maximum benefits and side effects. Over-the-counter preparations are also available, and they come as 60 mg capsules. You can take two of these three times a day and get the same benefit as the prescription strength.

Understanding all of that, here's what I usually recommend.

Orlistat can be taken by most people who want to begin a weight-loss program and will ultimately need pharmacologic help. This is the best place to start, since it's safe and effective. And if a person has diabetes or known cardiac risk factors, this will be a great choice.

I suggest that my patients try the OTC strength—60 mgs two or three times a day—and see how that works. They can increase this amount as tolerated. At the same time, I advise them to decrease their fat intake and increase their fiber. It's also important to begin taking a multivitamin, since several important fat-soluble vitamins can be lost through our GI tracts because of the increased fat excretion. Vitamin D is especially important here.

So orlistat is safe and effective. You can try this without risking any health hazards, and if you can overcome the potential side effects, it can be used long-term in your weight-loss efforts. While you can start this on your own with the OTC preparations, let your health-care provider know about it. This is still a team effort.

34

Prescription Weight-Loss Medicines, Part 2

Serotonin Activators

Remember fen-phen? This was a popular weight-loss product in the 1990s—a combination of fenfluramine and phentermine. Both of these medications were proven to be effective in weight loss—even more so when taken together.

The combo hit the market and sales rapidly escalated. Then serious medical problems began to be seen. Individuals taking fen-phen developed pulmonary hypertension—an increase in the blood pressure in the arteries, veins, and small vessels in the lungs. Symptoms included shortness of breath, fatigue, cough, chest pain, and dizziness. The treatments for this disorder are limited, and depending on the cause, a person's life-expectancy is significantly shortened, sometimes measured in just a few years.

The incidence of pulmonary hypertension skyrocketed, with estimates of between 25 and 50 million worldwide cases a year due to fen-phen. But which of these drugs was causing the problem? Phentermine has been around for a long time and has been relatively free of any major side effects. Certainly not pulmonary hypertension. And then we began to see heart-valve problems in this same group of people. Specifically, the mitral and aortic valves began to leak and fail, and people began to die. The drug was pulled from the market, and as it turns out, the manufacturer knew of these potential problems with the fenfluramine component yet failed to warn physicians or the public. As you can imagine, lawsuits totaling

billions of dollars continue to this day. Phentermine, the other component, was never proven to cause any of these heart or lung problems and
continues to be safely used for several medical conditions.

But what does this have to do with current weight-loss medications?
Fenfluramine was yanked off the market, right?

Right. The significance of this lies with fenfluramine's class of medication. It was a *serotonin activator*—a drug that acts on specific receptors
in the brain. When these receptors are stimulated, animals and humans
reduce their food intake and thus lose weight. This is a potentially valu-
able tool in our battle with obesity. The problem was that fenfluramine
was not very selective, and it activated some of the serotonin receptors that
reduced appetite but also were associated with the heart and lung problems noted above. Today we have at least one serotonin activator currently
being used for weight loss—lorcaserin. Its trade name is Belviq, and it is
a selective activator of a specific serotonin receptor and is a potent appetite suppressant. This specificity or selectiveness is supposed to make this
a safer drug than its predecessor, fenfluramine.

We know how this drug works, but how effective is it? How does it
compare to some of the other weight-loss drugs or even to a placebo?

The results seen with lorcaserin are consistently better than those with
a placebo (I'd hope so) and are about equal with what we discussed with
orlistat. As with orlistat, we see the additional benefits of a lower blood
pressure, reduced levels of total cholesterol and LDL, and better control
and even prevention of diabetes. All of these are probably related to the
loss of weight itself.

What about side effects? People on this drug won't experience the GI
problems associated with orlistat. But we're messin' with the brain here,
and frequent complaints include headache, dizziness, and nausea. In addition, back pain, upper respiratory infections, and sore throats are encountered. As many as one in five individuals on this drug will experience one
or several of these side effects, explaining why as many as 50 percent will
stop taking this medicine within 12 months.

So where does lorcaserin fit into a weight-loss program? Once again,
this is a drug, and we'll need to follow the same guidelines used for other
pharmacological interventions. There needs to be a failure to lose significant weight with lifestyle changes employed for at least six months (with
a BMI above 30) or with a BMI somewhere between 25 and 30 if at least

one obesity-related comorbidity is present. Then we'll need to make a choice as to the class or type of medication that should be used. As we noted with orlistat, that particular medication can safely be used by most people. With lorcaserin, this drug should not be used in the presence of significant kidney disease, in a pregnant or possibly pregnant woman, or with an array of other medications that act within the brain.

It's effective and can be considered when weight loss is critical for a person's well-being. I continue to be troubled by this class of medication—the serotonin activators. And while neither the incidence of heart-valve disease or pulmonary hypertension has been demonstrated to be statistically increased, both of these problems show a rising trend with use of this drug. That makes me nervous. It must make the FDA nervous as well. That regulatory organization requests ongoing trials to determine the long-term cardiovascular safety of this drug.

Time will tell. If you and your physician decide this might be a good choice for your weight-loss effort, make sure you know the facts. Both of you.

35

Prescription Weight-Loss Medicines, Part 3

The Stimulants

When weight-loss medicines are discussed, these are the ones most of us are thinking about. That's not surprising since far and away the number-one-selling weight-loss medicine is in this class—phentermine. You might know it as Adipex, Fastin, Ionamin, or some other name. And when it comes to the patients in our clinic, this is the medication most requested for weight loss.

Let's take a look at these stimulants and see what we know about them.

First, we know how these medicines work. They are all "centrally acting," meaning their site of action is within the brain. They stimulate nerve centers that tell us we're not hungry, and so we stop eating.

They are very effective in doing this, making them useful in our weight-loss efforts. This effectiveness is about the same as for the other types of medications, but no more so. Interestingly, since phentermine was first approved and released on the market in 1959, it didn't have to undergo the rigorous testing and proof of safety and efficacy that new drugs have to today. When we search the literature for solid evidence regarding these factors, it's just not there. Yet we know it works, and many physicians prescribe it—millions of times each year.

We also know that these stimulants are indicated only for short-term use—defined by most experts as 12 weeks or less. There are a couple of reasons for this. Very troubling is the potential for abuse with these or any drugs, hence the increased scrutiny regarding the prescribing practices of the stimulants. They are a type of "speed" and can easily fall into the wrong hands. That's why phentermine is a Schedule IV medication (not too far behind such drugs as Dilaudid, Demerol, Oxycontin, and Ritalin), indicating the seriousness of this problem and the need for close monitoring and the recommendation for short-term use.

The other reason for prescribing these medications for a brief time period is the risk profile associated with their use. All of these drugs will increase our heart rate and blood pressure, and they can cause dry mouth, constipation, insomnia, and nervousness. If that's not enough, other frequent side effects include dizziness, tremors, headache, and GI distress.

Because of these problems, many of us shouldn't take them. This group includes those who are pregnant or nursing, those with glaucoma, those with significant cardiovascular disease and uncontrolled hypertension, and those with hyperthyroidism. Additionally, if someone has a history of substance abuse, these medications should be avoided because of the abuse potential noted above.

These are significant concerns, and the use of the medications in this class should not be undertaken lightly. Consider the fate of previous stimulants:

- Sibutramine (Meridia) was taken off the European and US markets because of an increased risk of heart attacks and strokes.

- Phenylpropanolamine was taken off the US market because of a small but significant risk of strokes in women.

- Ephedrine (and its cousin Ephedra—commonly known as Ma Huang) has also been removed from the market because of an increased risk of irregular heartbeat, seizures, strokes, heart attacks, and death.

These are powerful drugs, and we have to ask ourselves where they should reasonably and responsibly be utilized in a weight-loss program. They are effective, and if used correctly, they can be safe. But we need to define *correctly*. This would include a careful screening for heart disease and some of the other problems listed above—thyroid disease, hypertension, and glaucoma. We also have to evaluate each individual's potential for abusing these medicines. And we need to limit the duration of treatment to 12 weeks, as directed by the FDA and experts in this field. You're probably not going to get this level of screening and scrutiny in a weight-loss clinic, and I recommend discussing any consideration of beginning one of these medicines with your regular health-care provider.

For completeness, we need to list the four currently available drugs in this class. We've already talked about phentermine, the most commonly prescribed. The other three are diethylpropion (Tenuate, Dospan), phendimetrazine (Bontril), and benzphetamine (Didrex). They are all "centrally acting," they all have the same side-effect concerns, and they are all about equally effective.

So that's what you need to know about the stimulants. In the hands of an experienced clinician and in the correct group of patients, these medications can be very effective in kick-starting meaningful weight loss. But *only* on a short-term basis.

36

Prescription Weight-Loss Medicines, Part 4

The Combinations

There are a couple of combination diet medications currently available, and we need to know something about them. The thought here is that if we combine two drugs with different mechanisms, we should be able to significantly enhance the weight-loss potential. We have a couple of these classes of drugs to choose from.

One class is the *antidepressants*. We've known for a while that some medications in this group are associated with weight loss, some with weight gain, and some are mainly neutral. The trick is to make this work to our advantage. Bupropion (Wellbutrin, Zyban) is one of the drugs that can cause weight loss. We learned this with its use in smoking cessation, finding that it could prevent the weight gain usually associated with this endeavor. It's actually a close relative of diethylpropion, one of the stimulant medications we discussed in an earlier chapter. Like its cousin, bupropion is thought to act in the brain, suppressing appetite. Weight loss with this drug alone has been associated with as much as a 5 to 7 percent loss of initial body weight over a six-month period.

The other class of medications currently in use in these combinations are those utilized for the control of seizures—the *antiepileptic drugs*. Seems a little unusual, but it's true. The one most of us are familiar with is topiramate (Topamax), which is used with seizures but also very commonly in the treatment of migraines. How it causes weight loss is not well understood. Some think it may be due to a decrease in saliva and loss of taste, thus making food less desirable. Others believe it exerts its effect through several hormonal pathways, including cortisol and insulin. There is also some evidence that it interferes with the blood level of leptin. But whatever the mechanism, topiramate is associated with an average weight loss of around 7 percent of baseline over a six-month period. Remember, our goal and the benchmark of a successful weight-loss effort is 5 percent over this span of time.

Now let's consider how some of our weight-loss medications are combined. The most commonly prescribed combination at this time is Qsymia (pronounced *kyoo-sim-EE-uh*—don't ask me), a combination of phentermine and topiramate. This drug was approved for use in 2012 and has the same indications as the other weight-loss medications—our BMI needs to be 30 or above, or 27 to 30 with at least one weight-related comorbidity. Since both of the medications in this combination can lead to weight loss, we would hope and expect that together we would experience greater success—and that turns out to be the case. For those who can take this medication, weight loss of 10 percent can be experienced. This will need to include a significant emphasis on lifestyle changes, but this kind of loss is impressive and significant.

But Qsymia isn't for everyone. Those with heart disease or uncontrolled high blood pressure and those who are or might become pregnant shouldn't take it. That still leaves many of us who might benefit from this medication.

"But doesn't this contain phentermine? I thought that was only for short-term use, not six months or more."

That's a great question, and I'm glad you were paying attention. You're right, the phentermine in this combination is generally for short-term use—up to 12 weeks. But Qsymia can be considered for longer periods of time because of the dosages involved. Most single phentermine preparations contain 37.5 mgs of active drug, while the amount in Qsymia starts at 7.5 mgs and maxes out at 15 mgs. The dosages of topiramate are also lower than when the drug is used by itself. All of this should help reduce the side effects of these medications, and it does. Yet as many as 20 percent of us taking this drug will experience problems, the most common of which are constipation, dry mouth, anxiety/depression, and tingling sensations in our hands and feet. Fortunately, most of these improve over the first few weeks of treatment.

This can be a helpful medication, but remember—it can't be used during pregnancy or in those who could potentially become pregnant, or in those of us with heart disease.

Another recent (2014) addition to the combination weight-loss drugs is Contrave. This medication contains bupropion and naltrexone. We've already mentioned how bupropion helps with weight loss. We also know it can be associated with an increased risk of depression and suicidal behavior, especially among teenagers and young adults. In this particular combination though, we haven't *yet* seen an increase in these problems.

The naltrexone component of this combination is an interesting drug. It acts within the brain at specific opioid sites, reducing our natural craving for food. Its side effects can include abdominal pain, rash, headache, joint pain, and fatigue. Chest pain, confusion, and hallucinations can occur, but these are rare. These side effects are bothersome enough that by the end of 12 months of treatment, only about 50 percent of individuals are still taking this medication.

Another difficulty with this medicine is its dosing schedule. A fairly elaborate ramp-up period is required, which might confuse many of us—it does me.

With all that said, just how effective is this combination? We can expect about a 4 to 5 percent loss of our baseline weight with Contrave. That's good, but we'll have to decide if the benefits of this medication outweigh the risks and side effects.

That's going to be the case with all of our combination weight-loss drugs. In fact, it's the case with any medication we're going to consider taking. Historically, several of these combinations are no longer on the market due to various complications and unforeseen problems. Time will tell about Qsymia and Contrave—and any of the other combos in the pipeline.

But there's one thing we can be sure of—and take to the bank. (The involved pharmaceutical companies certainly are.) There will be a huge market for any new medication that offers hope for weight loss. We just have to be armed with good information, a knowledgeable healthcare provider, and the certainty that if it sounds too good to be true, it probably is.

37

The HCG Diet

Are We Really Still Talking About This?

It never fails. At least once or twice a week, one of my patients will ask me what I think about these "new" HCG diets. It's usually someone who has tried everything—except diet and exercise—and has been unable to lose any weight. This is important for them to understand, so I pull up a chair, sit down, and this is what I tell them.

HCG (more correctly notated as hCG and known as the *human chorionic gonadotropin*) has been known to the scientific community for decades. It's a hormone produced by the placenta, and it has several important functions. In early pregnancy, its actions help nurture and sustain the growing embryo and help it implant itself in the uterine wall. The blood level of hCG rises predictably each day of pregnancy, allowing physicians to monitor the healthy progress of a normal pregnancy.

And it's the hormone measured in pregnancy tests, both over the counter and in a medical office or hospital. For those of us old enough to be familiar with the expression "the rabbit died" as indicating a positive pregnancy test, this same hCG was the culprit. In the 1930s, researchers determined that if the urine of a pregnant woman (containing high levels of hCG) was injected into a female rabbit, specific changes in the rabbit's ovaries would indicate the presence of hCG, and the woman would be found to be pregnant. Contrary to popular (and apparently persistent) opinion, the death of the rabbit didn't indicate a positive test. Rather, it was the changes noted in the ovaries, and the rabbit had to be sacrificed to examine them. We've come a long way, and Thumper (or his girlfriend) must be happy.

So that's hCG—a powerful hormone of pregnancy. But how did this ever become associated with weight loss? This is a good example of bad science gone worse.

Even if you're not a sports fan, you're probably familiar with the continuing controversy surrounding performance-enhancing drugs. We usually, and rightly, associate this with testosterone-like substances—hormones that promote the growth and strengthening of muscles. Many problems are encountered with these drugs. With prolonged use of these anabolic steroids, bothersome side effects can occur, including testicular atrophy. HCG has been found to counteract some of these effects and has made its way into this dangerous and illicit activity.

But prior to this, a British physician, Albert T.W. Simeons, developed a diet in the mid-1950s based on the use of hCG injections and an ultralow-calorie diet of only 500 calories. He claimed significant weight loss with no loss of muscle mass. P.T. Barnum would have known that if you rubbed snake oil on your belly and consumed no more than 500 calories each day, you were going to lose weight, and fast. But that amount of caloric restriction amounts to malnutrition, with its multiple and serious side effects. Scrutiny of Simeons's diet quickly debunked it, and over the ensuing years, multiple reputable agencies and organizations have attempted to place any hCG diet in its proper place.

Here's what the FDA had to say in 1976:

> The injection of HCG has not been approved by the Food and Drug Administration as safe and effective in the treatment of obesity or weight control. There is no substantial evidence that HCG increases weight loss beyond that resulting from caloric restriction.

And in 1995, the American Society of Bariatric Physicians took this position:

> There is no scientific evidence that HCG is effective in the treatment of obesity. The studies done to date have found insufficient evidence supporting the claims that HCG is effective in

altering fat-distribution, hunger reduction, or in inducing a feeling of well-being. The use of HCG should be regarded as an
inappropriate therapy for weight reduction.

Since that statement, no new studies refute this position or support
the use of hCG. And yet there are weight-loss clinics that tout its use and
seem to do a brisk business.

And then there's the Internet. I just went online and found the following advertisement of an amazing weight-loss product. Keep in mind that
you can lose "one to two pounds a day" and that this is "doctor approved."

HCG drops are taken orally [Interesting, since hCG is not
    absorbed through the GI tract]
No injections!
Same results as HCG clinics, but costs thousands of dollars
    less
No exercise needed while taking them
No prescription required
Our HCG has all-natural ingredients
No hunger pains while taking HCG diet drops
HCG converts fat into nutrients without loss of muscle

All of that sounds wonderful, doesn't it? And if you read a little farther,
you'll find more interesting information in the small print:

We are in compliance with the FDA guidelines since our for-
mulation doesn't contain the real HCG hormone, but only its
weight-reduction qualities.

Say what? And people actually buy this stuff?

So that's what I tell my patients. If they buy these products over the
counter or through the Internet, they're not getting real hCG. What's
actually in these bottles is anyone's guess. And if they're going to an "HCG
clinic" and getting the "real stuff," there are problems associated with these
injections. But mainly, it doesn't work, and you need to question the credentials and motivation of the practitioners in these clinics.

Save your money and stick with a reduced-calorie diet, but not as drastic as 500 calories.

38

Getting It Right

Isaac Dawkins

My partner and I had tried for years to get Isaac's attention.

"Isaac, you're a walking time bomb."

That exasperated warning from my partner had at least gotten the 58-year-old to throw away his cigarettes—no small feat. But when it came to addressing his other risk factors that were going to shorten his life, nothing seemed to work.

It had been six years since I informed him that he was a textbook example of the metabolic syndrome. He was at least 25 pounds overweight, his blood pressure remained elevated in spite of three maxed-out medications, his cholesterol and other lipids were out of control, and his blood sugar was always in the prediabetic range when we checked it. He couldn't help the fact that he was a male and over 50, but these other problems were things he could do something about. Or at least try.

"Doc, you can only do what you can do."

His wife, Sheila, was frustrated with him as well. When I mentioned keeping a food diary to help him get a handle on what he was eating and to lose some weight, she just laughed.

"Sure, Dr. Lesslie. Isaac might just as well bring in a copy of the *Betty Crocker Cookbook*."

And so it went. Each office visit became a predictable routine. Elevated blood pressure, a few pounds heavier, unhealthy lab work, and well-worn but entertaining excuses. We weren't making any progress.

Then Isaac missed a few appointments. No phone calls or emails. He just didn't show up for his scheduled office visits. Our nurses tried to contact him but were never successful.

"We've got a work-in." Sarah, our lead nurse, stood beside me, holding a patient's folder.

I glanced at my watch—12:30. My lunch break, scheduled for noon, was almost over, and I had yet to sit down. The morning had been busy, and we were running late. I sighed and shook my head.

"I think you'll want to see this one."

Isaac Dawkins sat on the exam table of room 3, his wife standing at his side.

"It's been a while, Isaac." I opened his chart and thumbed to today's office notes.

"Over a year," his wife said, her voice unsmiling.

"It's like I always said, Doc, if you don't make any changes, what's the use of coming in? I hadn't been making any changes—not until recently. And now it's time to come in to see you."

I looked at his weight and then flipped to his last visit. Isaac had been 230 pounds a year ago, and now weighed...35 pounds less. And today his blood pressure was perfect—118/78. He had come to the office a few days earlier for fasting lab work, and I turned to that report. His blood sugar was perfect, and his cholesterol and triglycerides were now normal. Even his HDL—the good cholesterol—was in a healthy range.

I stared at him. "Isaac, how did you do this?"

"Do what? The weight you mean? Oh, I just did some of the things you told me. Some of the things you probably thought I wasn't payin' any attention to. I started keeping that diary you always said to do, and I was amazed at the amount of junk I was eating. Then I tried that Atkins thing, the low-carb diet. That part was easy, and I lost about ten pounds over the first month or so. Then things just stopped, and I started exercising more. Sheila and I started walking every evening, for at least 45 minutes, sometimes more. She's lost some weight too."

Isaac paused and beamed at his wife.

"But the weight wouldn't come off, and I knew I had to try something.

I did some readin' and went to the drugstore and bought some of that over-the-counter stuff, orlistat I think it's called. It's supposed to keep you from absorbing fat, and I thought that made sense. But there were some side effects…"

Sheila looked down and shook her head.

"But it was workin'," Isaac continued. "So I did some more readin' and found out that if you cut down on the amount of fat you're eating, those side effects usually go away. And they did. Eatin' less fat makes sense too. And the weight started dropping again. I got down to my target—even a little lower—and decided it was time to come see you, and see what my blood sugar and other stuff was doin'."

"They're doing great, Isaac. And so is your blood pressure. And 195 pounds…That's impressive. You *were* listening to what we've been talking about."

"Well, Sheila was doin' most of the listenin' and most of the coachin'. I couldn't have done this without her help."

"It takes a team, doesn't it?" I agreed. "And it looks like you've got a good coach. So that's the *how* of your weight loss and everything else, but tell me about the *why*. What finally prompted you to do this? I know it wasn't our constant nagging."

"Well, no it wasn't." Isaac shifted on the table and reached for the wallet in his back pocket. He took out a small, wrinkled photo and handed it to me.

Isaac Dawkins was standing in front of a chain-link fence, wearing a baseball cap and grinning from ear to ear. He was flanked by two small boys, probably five or six years old, both dressed in baseball uniforms. They weren't looking at the camera, but up at the man standing between them.

"Your grandsons?"

Isaac smiled.

"The rest of my team."

39

Commercial Weight-Loss Plans

Do They Work and Are They Worth It?

I was skeptical as I began doing research for this topic. After all, ready-made meals arriving at your doorstep may be a marketing success, but I had my doubts as to how this could reasonably fit into a sound and successful weight-loss effort. However, I felt it needed to be included in any book that tried to responsibly cover the broad subject of weight loss. I also must clearly state that I have no vested interest in any of these plans or companies, and my intention is simply to provide you with the most accurate and up-to-date information I can find.

Fortunately, I found a recent article in the *Annals of Internal Medicine* that sheds light on this subject. This is a well-respected medical journal, and the authors of this research studied the available literature and pulled together more than 40 studies, most of them randomized control trials (RCTs). This is the most sophisticated and reliable method of studying health questions and is considered the gold standard for clinical trials. These were not anecdotal cases or small studies of questionable methodology. The information here should be reliable.

The study started from the position that since commercial weight-loss programs were becoming more popular and pervasive, the question of their benefit should be established. The authors looked at studies of the more commonly encountered products that compared them to control

groups. These control groups were weight-loss efforts that included counseling and caloric restriction without a specified dietary plan. In other
words, they tried as much as possible to compare apples to apples, with
the variable being the commercial program's diet and approach to counseling. Here's what they found:

- By the end of 12 months, those using Weight Watchers
  achieved at least 2.6 percent greater weight loss than controls.

- By 12 months, individuals in the Jenny Craig program experienced at least 4.9 percent greater loss.

- The studies with Nutrisystem were of shorter duration—only
  about 3 months—but the results were around a 4 percent
  advantage compared to controls.

Other proprietary weight-loss programs were evaluated, but the studies were usually of shorter duration and demonstrated mixed results.
The authors of this report concluded:

- Physicians could consider referring their patients who are
  in need of weight loss to Jenny Craig or Weight Watchers. Nutrisystem can be a consideration, but further studies,
  including long-term results, are needed.

- Participation in these programs should be short-term only
  (about a year), with a significant emphasis on lifestyle
  changes. Effective personal counseling is considered a key
  component for a sustained weight-loss program.

I found these results and recommendations interesting, and not necessarily what I expected. It's caused me to take a closer look at these programs and to consider recommending them for some of my patients. The
most appropriate use of these would be for individuals who do best with
a very structured dietary plan and who might have trouble finding effective weight-loss counseling. As noted, these plans should be viewed as a
bridge, with lifestyle changes, portion control, and food choices being the
resultant benefits.

Now let's take a look at each of these three programs.

40

Jenny Craig

The Jenny Craig Company was founded in Australia in 1983 by Jenny Craig and her husband, Sidney (not to be confused with Sydney). Since then, they have expanded their operations around the world and in this country. In the United States, they're headquartered in California.

This weight-loss program combines individual weight-management counseling with a menu of frozen meals and various other foods. Orders are placed, and these meals can be directly shipped to your home or picked up at designated centers. In addition, there are several specialized plans to choose from, including for elderly individuals, for those with diabetes, and for those who prefer a meatless diet.

The key component here is the counseling, with its emphasis on lifestyle changes. This includes eating habits, exercise, and nutritional education. Counseling is purportedly provided through private, individual sessions. The counselors, while trained by the company, are not necessarily certified health professionals. As mentioned in our chapter on the behavioral management of weight loss, this counseling is an important and integral part of any successful program. Several of my patients have tried this system but neglected to take part in the counseling. They lost some weight at first, but plateaued after a couple of weeks and then gave up. If you're going to try the Jenny Craig program, make sure you avail yourself of this service.

The program claims to follow the current USDA dietary guidelines, stressing the inclusion of vegetables, fruits, lean meat, fish, eggs, and nuts, while reducing or eliminating salt, added sugars, cholesterol, and saturated fats. Still, those with high blood pressure will need to examine the food labels for sodium content, and diabetics will need to monitor the amount of carbs they're consuming.

The stated mission is to help individuals reach their weight-loss goal, educate them to appropriate lifestyle changes, teach them sound nutritional principles, and equip them to maintain their new weight. Though these changes and goals are appropriate and achievable, the purchase of the Jenny Craig food plan should be limited to no more than one year. If you're going to try this program, keep that in mind. And make sure you participate in the weight-management counseling.

For more information, visit www.jennycraig.com.

41

Weight Watchers

Weight Watchers International (WW) tips the scales at $1.72 billion in sales (reported in 2013). That's pretty impressive, and the company is listed and publicly traded on the New York Stock Exchange (its symbol is WTW). WW was founded in 1963 by a homemaker living in Queens, New York—Jean Nidetch. The company now operates in 30 countries around the world, with Oprah Winfrey being a significant stockholder (listed as 10 percent).

Their approach is different from most of the other commercial weight-loss programs in that the current emphasis of WW is not about supplying food products to its clients. Rather, the focus is on helping people lose weight by eating smarter, forming helpful habits and overcoming bad ones, getting more exercise, and providing ongoing support. They try to do this with something called the OnlinePlus plan, currently the primary plan offered in the United States. This assigns points for just about every type and variety of food. A calculation is made based on the client's individual needs and weight-loss goal, and then a points total is assigned. The focus is on reducing overall caloric intake, and if the participant is able to stay within this point total, weight loss has been demonstrated to occur.

This technique requires dedication and discipline. A person in the program has to understand the point system and be willing to regularly keep up with it. But again, if this is done, the plan works. As an aside, the tracking tools of this program can easily be applied to other reduced-calorie diets and strategies, further improving the chances of a successful outcome.

WW encourages increased physical activity and rewards this behavior by allowing clients to add points to their daily total, based on defined types and amounts of various exercises and activities.

And since it is generally agreed that counseling and support are important for any successful program, WW holds meetings for its members in many locations, providing that support and reinforcement. In fact, they claim that participants who use the point-counting tools *and* attend these meetings increase their potential for weight loss and for achieving their goal. Included in these meetings is an emphasis on healthy eating and breaking poor dietary habits. While researching this program, I came across an interesting term: *hedonic hunger*. WW apparently defines this as "the desire to seek out high-sugar, high-fat foods that bring pleasure." Avoiding hedonic hunger is a lofty and worthy goal, but easier said than done.

While we mentioned that the provision of prepackaged food was not the main emphasis of WW, this might be changing. The company is branching out into food products as well as cookbooks, DVDs, and even exercise equipment. Interestingly, the H.J. Heinz Company, one of the early owners of WW, continues to supply packaged foods for the brand.

In summary, Weight Watchers provides a proven framework for restructuring how much and what we eat. Their elaborate system won't be for everyone, but for those who can faithfully and honestly keep up with their points, it works. We know that's true for up to 12 months, but beyond that amount of time, there are no reputable studies that demonstrate ongoing success and weight maintenance.

One of the positive long-term by-products of this program may turn out to be the mental and emotional adjustments that happen when dealing with this point system. That should give us an appreciation for the relative value of various foods and the importance of portion size. And that is what it takes for lifelong dietary changes.

For more information, visit www.weightwatchers.com.

42

Nutrisystem

Of the three commercial weight-loss programs we're considering, Nutri-sytem is the latest to gain a significant market presence. It has changed through the years, moving from being largely a brick-and-mortar company to an online, direct-to-consumer model. This has had a significant impact on what they can offer their clients, especially as it relates to the availability of face-to-face personal counseling.

Nutrisystem bases its approach to weight loss on the established fact that using a structured low-calorie diet improves the chances of weight loss when compared to an individual choosing his or her own diet. They do this by structured meal plans and attention to portion control. As mentioned earlier, current information indicates that this tactic is successful, at least in the short term (about three months). There are no studies that demonstrate continued weight loss or maintenance of lost weight beyond that time period.

Nutrisystem offers more than 150 menu choices for breakfast, lunch, dinner, and snacks/desserts. These products don't supply all of a client's dietary needs—only about 60 percent. The remainder comes from foods bought at the grocery store, with guidance from the company. These include fresh fruits and vegetables, various proteins, and low-fat dairy items.

The plan's diet implements a low-calorie approach as well as a focus on foods with a low glycemic index. Foods with a high glycemic index would be things such as sugar, a baked potato, waffles, and even corn flakes—foods that require a burst of insulin to handle and that challenge our pancreas. Eliminating these high glycemic index foods is a good idea, especially for those of us with borderline or full-blown diabetes.

That part makes sense. But the rap against Nutrisystem has been that the plan doesn't foster and support long-term weight control. The concern is that an individual may have success while using the company's calorie-controlled prepackaged foods, but once that ends, any benefits will soon be lost. The company has responded by trying to implement more counseling and support for its clients and encouraging more physical activity. This may prove difficult, since Nutrisystem has no clinics or centers to provide face-to-face interactions. We'll have to see how that turns out, and whether long-term studies will show continued success with this weight-loss plan.

For more information, visit www.nutrisystem.com.

As I stated from the outset, I have no vested interest in any of these companies, and if asked to choose one over the other two, I would decline to do so. I won't recommend any of these plans to the majority of my patients. Some patients will benefit from a more structured dietary plan, and for these I would discuss their options. The bottom line with the use of any of these is to consider it only as a bridge, coupling its use with significant lifestyle changes. Some of these programs are aggressive with their counseling, and that's a good thing. Others seem to leave their clients more on their own, which doesn't lend itself to a successful outcome.

Some of the tools for self-monitoring (Weight Watchers, as an example) can be very helpful and instructive. That's a real plus for any weight-loss effort. Portion control (Jenny Craig and Nutrisystem) is also vital for long-term weight management. So if I sound ambivalent here, I suppose I am.

If you're intent on trying one of these programs, be sure you know what you're getting into and the financial investment you're going to make. Twelve months is the maximum amount of time to rely on their food products. From the outset, you can't rely only on their system to achieve your goal. You have to pay attention to lifestyle changes, and you need to access whatever counseling they make available—and do so regularly.

These programs can be a start. But they won't be the finish.

43

Bariatric Surgery, Part 1

What Are We Talking About?

Let's start with the word *bariatric*. When I was in medical school and for a couple of decades beyond, I hadn't heard much of this term. It's relatively new—beginning to come into use around 1965. It's now firmly attached to the field of weight loss (some would say "industry"). The Greek root here—*baro* or *baros*—means "weight," and *iatric* means "treatment." Simple enough. So now we have the expanding (no pun intended) scope of bariatric treatments.

Some of these treatments include the surgical approach to excessive or morbid obesity. Remember your BMI chart. This would be in the zone above 40, and that will be important.

In the mid-1950s, a surgeon by the name of A.J. Kremen performed some of the first bariatric surgeries. The initial procedure was to divide the small intestine and remove a significant portion of it. The upper section was then linked to the lower part. This significantly shortened the normally 23 feet of the small intestine, where most of our digestive absorption takes place. The remaining unused section was discarded. The theory behind this intestinal bypass was that if you eliminated most of the small intestine, you would reduce the amount of nutrients and calories absorbed into the bloodstream and body. It worked—maybe too well. Complications were frequent and included dehydration, vitamin deficiencies, electrolyte abnormalities (sodium, potassium, chloride) and a bothersome and embarrassing chronic diarrhea.

The weight loss was impressive, though, and the medical community knew the surgeons were on to something. The key would be to find a procedure that was effective in causing weight loss but also safe.

Over the next few decades, this area of surgery became more refined, and the techniques and procedures became easier to perform and much safer. The concept is simple—decrease the absorption of nutrients and increase the feeling of being full. In the next chapter, we'll take a look at the most common of these approaches, how they work, and which ones might be right for specific types of people. For right now, though, just keep in mind that about eight different bariatric surgical approaches are performed in the United States today.

And these surgeries are performed a lot. In 2011, more than 350,000 of these procedures were done in the United States alone. That number seems to have stabilized around the 200,000 per year mark, thought to be due to an improving success rate of nonsurgical weight loss with a comprehensive, team-based approach. Yet many of us will need to consider bariatric surgery if we are to ever achieve a more normal weight.

This is where our BMI comes into play again. In order to be an appropriate candidate for bariatric surgery, a person's BMI needs to exceed 40, or be higher than 35 or so with the presence of obesity-related comorbidities. Let's consider those for a moment, because the list is longer than you might think. Here are some of the serious comorbidities, of which the presence of at least one will qualify a person for bariatric surgery:

- type 2 diabetes
- elevated/abnormal lipids (cholesterol)
- obstructive sleep apnea
- asthma
- gastroesophageal reflux disease (GERD)
- high blood pressure
- nonalcoholic fatty liver disease
- debilitating arthritis
- impaired quality of life

- severe urinary incontinence
- certain causes of increased intracranial pressure
- diseases of the veins

We noted that if a person's BMI was greater than 35 and they had one of these problems, that combination would qualify them for this surgery. That number of 35 is lowered to 30 in the presence of uncontrollable type 2 diabetes or the metabolic syndrome, which we've already looked at. These issues are so serious that it's imperative to get them under control. And bariatric surgery has been proven to help.

That's a long list, and it turns out to fit a lot of us. And as we've seen, the number in the over-40 zone of the BMI chart, as well as the number of people with these diseases, continues to grow—meaning that more and more of us will be qualifying for these procedures.

But there are a few things that will usually prevent an individual from being qualified by a responsible surgeon (and approved by insurance companies). First is the consideration of age. Most of us who are younger than 18 or older than 65 would not be approved. This is not ironclad and would be determined on a case-by-case basis. Other things that will knock us off the "accepted" list are:

- current alcohol or drug abuse
- untreated major depression or psychosis
- uncontrolled and untreated eating disorders
- severe bleeding problems
- the inability to maintain lifelong nutritional requirements either from an established medical problem or a psychological disorder
- severe heart disease with significant surgical risks

So with all this in mind, who are some people who have had this type of surgery? Maybe some of your friends and family. But how about this list:

Brian Dennehy	Randy Jackson (of *American Idol* fame)
Roseanne Barr	Rex Ryan (NFL coach)

John Daly (golfer)	Chris Christie (New Jersey governor)
Rosie O'Donnell	Jessie Jackson Jr.
Etta James	Sharon Osbourne

And more than a million others. If you're considering this surgery, or have been advised to do so by your physician, what can you expect? How much weight loss might be possible if you elect to have one of these procedures? The answer turns out to be a lot. Somewhere between 50 and 70 percent of a person's current weight—more than *half* of an individual's size! And in the right hands, it can happen safely and quickly. But how safely and how quickly?

In the next couple of chapters, we'll answer those questions and lay out a clear course for those of us navigating the waters of this sometimes confusing issue.

44

Bariatric Surgery, Part 2

What Are Our Choices?

We've considered the history and development of weight-loss surgery and understand that this field of medicine, while maturing, is still in a state of refinement and a little flux. There are several types of procedures to choose from, depending on our particular needs, circumstances, and even where we live, and we need to have a clear understanding of what they involve. We have to understand the indications, costs, and risks.

Before deciding on a specific type of surgery, your surgeon, or the healthcare facility, you first need to ask, what does the overall weight-loss program look like? The surgical procedure itself should never occur as an isolated event, but rather be supported by an effective multidisciplinary team of professionals. These should include individuals with expertise in nutrition and exercise, psychological counselors, and lifestyle-modification coaches. A plan and ongoing program must be in place before you are ever wheeled into an operating room. Most reputable facilities that offer weight-loss surgery will have this team in place, but you have to ask.

This is a life-changing experience and a lifelong commitment. And the reality is that if we find ourselves in the over-40 BMI range, we got there on our own. But the odds are against us in ever getting out of that range without help and long-term assistance.

So how do these surgeries work? There are two basic mechanisms by which these procedures allow us to lose weight: decreased absorption of nutrients/energy, and something called *restriction*—a smaller stomach. Pretty simple stuff when you think about it—decreased absorption of calories or a smaller stomach that causes us to more quickly feel full. A growing body of evidence suggests that other factors are at play here, such as the alteration of hormones and other chemicals that affect how much and how often we eat, as well as how we handle the nutrients that are absorbed into our systems. This is interesting information, and we'll consider this later on.

Most surgical procedures fall into one of these categories—restriction or decreased absorption (we'll refer to this as *malabsorption*), but there are a couple of instances where both will be involved. Let's start with the restrictive surgeries, since they are simpler and less involved than the malabsorptive ones.

The restrictive surgeries limit the intake of calories by reducing the size of the stomach. A normal stomach can expand to accommodate as much as 1000 milliliters (about 32 ounces or 4 cups). Some of these surgeries will reduce this capacity to 30 milliliters (about 2 tablespoons). That's not much, and we can understand how that feeling of fullness can quickly develop in this setting. There are several types of these procedures, including the laparoscopic adjustable gastric band (LAGB), the vertical banded gastroplasty (VBG), and the sleeve gastrectomy. Figures 1 and 2 demonstrate the LAGB and the sleeve approaches, giving us an easy-to-understand visualization of what's going on here.

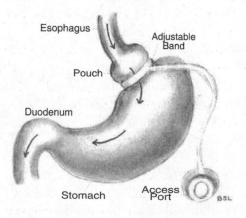

Figure 1   Gastric Banding

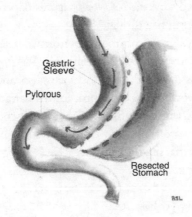

Figure 2   Sleeve Gastrectomy

It's really very simple—all of these restrictive surgeries *restrict* the size of the stomach, thereby reducing the amount of food we can eat at one time, leading to weight loss. With the LAGB, a tight adjustable band is placed around the entrance to the stomach. The adjustment can take place by inflating or deflating a bulb located just below the skin and accessed with a needle and syringe. The gastric sleeve involves removal of a large part of the stomach, with multiple staples closing the incision left behind in the greatly reduced stomach. The weight loss associated with these surgeries is more gradual than we find with the malabsorptive procedures, which turn out to be more complex to perform.

These purely malabsorption procedures, the surgeries that reduce the absorption of nutrients, do so by reducing the length of the small intestine (where the majority of our food absorption takes place). This is done in a couple of ways—either surgically removing part of the small intestine or diverting around (bypassing) a significant part of it. These surgeries can result in extreme weight loss, but can also produce significant metabolic complications by the disruption of needed calories, vitamins, minerals, and other essential nutrients. Most of these procedures are no longer performed because of the many complications associated with them. A couple of examples are the *jejunoileal bypass* and the *biliopancreatic diversion.* Doesn't sound like much fun, and it wasn't. Their disappearance from the commonly performed surgeries for weight loss is part of that refinement and maturing we mentioned earlier.

This brings us to the most commonly performed weight-loss surgery—the Roux (pronounced *roo*) -en-Y gastric bypass (RYGB). Figure 3 will be helpful as we discuss this procedure. (You can also find a video demonstration at www.mayoclinic.org/tests-procedures/bariatric-surgery/multimedia/gastric-bypass/vid-20084648.) It's the most common because it works, we know what to expect with it, and we can manage the anticipated complications that might develop.

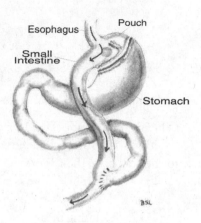

Figure 3   Roux-en-Y Gastric Bypass

This is a combination procedure in that it combines both a restrictive element (the smaller stomach pouch) with a much-shortened small intestine, thus providing a malabsorption component.

Whew, that's a mouthful. But after all, that's what we're trying to cut down on—the mouthfuls. Each of these approaches can lead to significant and lifesaving weight loss—most in the range of 5 to 70 percent of initial body weight. There are other less frequently used surgeries out there, but these are the most common.

And there are some experimental procedures as well. One of these includes the use of a soft, saline-filled balloon placed inside the stomach to give us a feeling of being full without eating too much. Another involves blocking the impulses from the vagal nerves with electrical stimulation from an implanted device. Blocking these important nerves interferes with messages sent from the stomach to the brain, thus reducing the feeling of hunger. This is purely investigational at present, so we'll just have to see. And then there's the mini-gastric bypass, an abbreviated modification of the RYGB. It's easier to perform (usually laparoscopically) but is associated with some serious complications that will have to be overcome before its use becomes widespread.

So those are the bariatric surgeries we'll encounter as we consider this area of weight-loss intervention. Most are very safe and effective, and if it's necessary and you're in the right hands, it's something that shouldn't be feared.

This is a good time to mention *liposuction*. While most of us view this as a cosmetic surgical procedure, some (with the help of some of the surgeons who perform it) think of it as a good way to lose weight. It is true that if you remove a substantial amount of fatty tissue, you're going to lose weight. But frequently it is regained since there is no multidisciplinary approach to encourage ongoing lifestyle changes. And the purported benefits of improving the control of type 2 diabetes and abnormal cholesterol levels just aren't true.

If you want to remove fat from specific areas, liposuction may be for you. If you really need to lose a lot of weight, modify your risk factors, and potentially save your life, you know where to turn—bariatric surgery.

45

Bariatric Surgery, Part 3

The Pros, the Cons, and What You Can Expect

We've already mentioned that bariatric surgery can result in as much as a 50 to 70 percent total body weight loss. Nothing else can approach that kind of outcome, and in many people, this can be lifesaving. For those with BMIs greater than 40 and who undergo one of these surgeries, their near and long-term death rates (from all causes) can be reduced by as much as 40 percent. That's big.

How does this happen? As you would expect, with successful surgery and adherence to an overall lifestyle improvement plan, many comorbidities substantially improve or simply go away. What are some of the things we're talking about here?

Let's start with high blood pressure. As many as 70 percent of those with hypertension are able to completely stop their medications. And for the remaining 30 percent, they are usually able to reduce the number and dosage of whatever medicines are required. That spells financial savings and fewer side effects.

Type 2 diabetes (adult onset) can be reversed in as many as 90 percent of people—90 percent! That's amazing, but that's the number. A normal blood sugar and no more medications. But how fast does this happen? Usually in a matter of weeks, but sometimes days. That's great news for many of us, but it's something we need to watch closely as it can be a short-term liability—a dangerously low blood sugar can quickly develop. This can be anticipated and easily prevented.

Elevated lipid levels (cholesterol, LDL, triglycerides) can be corrected in almost three out of four people who have this problem. More monetary savings and fewer side effects. An interesting and recently developing point here is that while all forms of bariatric surgery improve lipid abnormalities, gastric bypass is associated with the greatest and most consistent lowering of LDL—the "bad cholesterol" that we believe is most responsible for the development of heart disease and other vascular problems. Something to keep in mind when we recommend a specific type of surgery for a specific patient.

Obstructive sleep apnea frequently goes away, thus allowing many individuals to throw away their CPAP machines (making it a lot easier to get through security at the airport). Keep in mind that obesity is the leading cause of sleep problems in the first place.

Most studies demonstrate that low-back and joint pain is relieved in almost all people after this surgery. That is helped by the ability to increase aerobic exercise, such as walking or swimming.

And while we mentioned the decrease in mortality (all causes of death) among those having these procedures, we need to put a finer point on this. The most current information indicates that those who have a bariatric procedure will have a 90 percent reduction in their risk of dying over the five years following their surgery than if they didn't have the surgery. Again, that's a big and important number.

So we know that this surgery works and that it really helps people. But are there drawbacks? Is there a downside, and if so, what is it?

Most silver linings have a cloud, and bariatric surgery is no exception. There are some problems to be expected, many of which can be prevented with preparation and ongoing vigilance. Let's start with the procedure itself.

As with all surgical operations, there is an unavoidable risk of injury or even death. Most experts place the chances of postoperative complications with bariatric surgery in the 0 to 15 percent range. Most of these will resolve over days or weeks and not cause any long-term problem. One long-term problem is the possibility of death, and in the best centers, this number maxes out at about 0.5 percent of patients undergoing the most invasive and complicated surgery—gastric bypass. That's about 1 death out of every 200 cases. How does this compare with other surgeries? Here are some estimates, keeping in mind that accurate data is hard to come by and varies from region to region and across ages, genders, and races.

appendectomy—1/1200
cardiac bypass—1/30
mitral valve surgery—1/7
tummy tuck—1/600
facelift—1/1000
C-section—1/1000
normal vaginal delivery—1/10,000

That gives us an idea of where the risk of gastric bypass falls in comparison to other commonly performed surgeries. And keep in mind, the gastric bypass procedures carry the most risk of the various bariatric surgeries, with the other types being safer.

Now we need to consider the specifics of these potential complications. First, there are the problems encountered with any invasive abdominal procedure.

Bleeding. The stomach is a vascular organ with many blood vessels. A lot of these vessels have to be cut in order to perform the surgery and can be a source of rebleeding. A lot of blood can be lost during the operation, requiring potential transfusions.

Infection. This complication can involve the skin incision or deeper layers of the abdominal wall. When an infection spreads to the inside of the abdominal cavity, we have real problems. Good surgical technique will prevent most of these infections, but anytime you incise the stomach or intestinal tract, the potential for bacterial contamination is present.

Blood clots. This is always a risk with any surgery. The concern here is for the clots that form in the legs and then move up into the lungs—the deadly pulmonary embolism. Blood thinners are effective in preventing and treating this complication.

Hernias. A hernia is an abnormal weakness or opening through the abdominal wall muscles. It can occur almost anywhere, and can happen after any surgical procedure. Complications can include a simple but unsightly bulging at the site of the surgery, or a dangerous internal hernia that can result in a bowel obstruction.

Intestinal obstruction. And speaking of bowel obstruction, this can happen anytime the insides of our bellies are manipulated. Scarring can occur (adhesions), leading to a twisting of the small intestine or other organ around the adhesion and resultant blockage. If this happens, we're going to know it—pain, vomiting, fever. One of the problems with this type of complication is that it can occur months and even years after the surgery. Something to think about if you've ever had any surgical procedure.

Okay, is that enough to make you want to stay out of the operating room? Wait, we're not finished. There are some complications specific to gastric bypass procedures.

First we have something called an *anastomotic stricture.* This occurs at the site where two ends of intestine are put back together. Scar tissue normally forms there, and when it becomes too tight, the passage becomes smaller and smaller. This can result in pain and even an obstruction. Fortunately the fix is relatively simple and involves placing a balloon inside the stricture and inflating it until an acceptable amount of expansion has been restored. This is the same thing that happens when a stent is placed in a diseased and blocked coronary artery.

Leakage can also happen at the *anastomosis.* The seal between the two ends of intestine might break down or might not have been watertight at the time of surgery. This is serious, and unless the leak is minor and quickly resolves on its own, a reoperation will need to take place.

If that were not enough, an *ulcer* can develop at this same location. This happens in as many as 15 percent of patients having gastric bypass. This occurs for a lot of reasons, including increased levels of gastric acid, reduced local blood flow, and even smoking. The treatment is straightforward and includes medications and a reduction in solid food.

In addition to these surgical complications, many nutritional problems can develop, including iron deficiency (common signs include fatigue, depression, mouth and tongue lesions, and headaches), zinc deficiency (hair loss, depression, white spots on the fingernails), various B-vitamin deficiencies, and the development of a negative protein balance. These complications can be prevented with anticipation and the early and continued use of supplements and dietary manipulation. We know a lot about these now, and they can almost always be prevented.

That's a long list of bad stuff, and we have to wonder if this could possibly be worth the potential dangers. Can the benefits of this surgery ever outweigh the risks? The answer is almost always yes.

But here's something to keep in mind and to ask your potential surgeon. How many operations has he or she performed? That's a good question before any serious procedure. The old medical school adage of "see one, do one, teach one" doesn't apply here. Conventional wisdom tells us that the magic number for proficiency is at least 100 successful bariatric surgeries. Ask for a specific number, and if it's not at least 100, say thank you and look for another surgeon. The same holds true for the hospital where this might be performed. Ask about their experience with bariatric surgery and about their complication rates. If they stutter and stammer, it's time to get back in your car and head elsewhere.

So now we know the benefits of these surgeries, for whom they're intended, and the things we need to be looking out for. And we know the questions we need to ask if our physician recommends we pursue this path. That's a good start.

Choosing a Bariatric Surgeon

Does It Make a Difference?

You know the answer to this question—of course it does. But how do we go about making an informed decision? And maybe just as important, how do we decide where we want to have the procedure performed? These are two significant questions, and most of us will need some help in answering them. Fortunately, there are several good sources for guidance.

A good place to start is with our primary care physician. He or she should be guiding us in our weight-loss journey and should be able to advise us regarding the need and advisability of having bariatric surgery. Not all family practitioners are versed in this area, but it's a reasonable place to start.

Once we've started this discussion, several steps will need to be taken. By this time, our knowledge of the importance of diet, exercise, and counseling should be secure, and these lifestyle modifications should be in place. And then we need to have an understanding of the various surgical procedures available to us, the potential complications, and what we can reasonably expect as the upside. The last couple of chapters should have prepared us for the next step, which is to begin our search for potential bariatric doctors and bariatric weight-loss centers. We'll start with selecting the surgeon.

Only a few years ago, many general surgeons began to branch out into weight-loss surgery. A Monday morning schedule might include a hernia repair, gall-bladder removal, and then a weight-loss procedure squeezed in before lunch. This is still going on in some parts of the country, but it's something to avoid. This is complicated surgery, performed on complicated patients with complicated problems. We want our surgeon to know what he or she is doing; we don't want him or her performing bariatric surgery simply as a new service line.

Determining the qualifications of a potential surgeon is not difficult. First, they need to be actively and fully licensed to practice medicine in their state. And they need to be board certified in their specialty—typically general surgery. This certification requires a demonstrable level of expertise and commitment as well as ongoing medical education.

But that's not enough. We want our surgeon to have the appropriate credentials for performing weight-loss surgery. He or she should participate in organizations such as the American Society for Metabolic and Bariatric Surgeons (ASMBS). This same organization confers the designation of BSCOE (Bariatric Surgery Center of Excellence) to surgeons who perform at least 50 bariatric procedures each year (with a minimum of 125 such surgeries in their lifetime). This is important. The more bariatric surgeries a physician performs, the more proficient they become, and the more capable they become in handling the complications that will predictably arise. Both experience and research indicate that for every 10 bariatric procedures each year above that threshold of 50 cases, the risk of complications goes down by 10 percent. Once again, we don't want our surgery performed by a part-time weight-loss surgeon and sandwiched between a couple of hernia repairs.

What about the location of our surgery? What hospitals or medical centers should we consider? The ASMBS can help us here as well. They credential hospitals as being a Center of Excellence (COE) based on several factors. First, the facility has to perform at least 125 bariatric procedures each year. And second, they have to have in place a comprehensive multidisciplinary team that supports their surgical patients. This team should stress all the lifestyle changes we've been discussing and it should become involved long before we're put to sleep for the surgery. In addition, any potential medical complications will need to be evaluated and addressed.

Members of this team should include a bariatric program director, psychologist, dietitian or nutritionist, and fitness advisor. As the day of surgery approaches, the group will expand to include an insurance coordinator (this is an important consideration not to be overlooked), an anesthesiologist, and potentially lung and heart specialists. A support team of counselors and previous patients should already be in place, since we know that those who regularly attend support groups have better long-term outcomes.

And regarding outcomes, all hospitals and surgeons who have earned the accreditation of being BSCOE are required to give a detailed report of their patients' outcomes. This is something called BOLD (Bariatric Outcomes Longitudinal Database) and provides a way to keep an eye on bariatric physicians and centers and to monitor for any red flags that might pop up.

Sounds like a lot to do, and it is. But if we're going to consider having this surgery, we want to be sure we have the best possible chances of success. A little homework in selecting the right surgeon and medical center will yield positive results and peace of mind.

For more information about choosing a qualified surgeon and bariatric surgical facility, try these websites:

www.obesityaction.org
http://asmbs.org/
http://mbsaqip.org/

47

Getting It Right

The Tortoise and the Hare

Jerry Rogers sat on the edge of the exam table and beamed.

"Doc, I've got some great news. And I need to thank you."

I pulled up a chair and opened the 56-year-old's medical record. We had been treating his blood pressure and elevated cholesterol for more than ten years, and on his last visit these, as always, were under control. *What could be his good news?*

"It's my weight."

I glanced at the chart again, flipping the pages to his visit six months earlier—196 pounds. Today he weighed 182. That was impressive. We had talked about the importance of losing weight as a way to control his blood pressure and get his lipids under control. And his strong family history of diabetes was even more reason to aggressively lower his BMI—which at 196 pounds put him above 36.

"This is great, Jerry. Tell me how you did it."

"It's not so much *how* I did it, Doc, it's *why* I did it. I guess it all flows together though, so I'll tell you *how* first. All I did was follow the advice you gave me. First I came up with a goal—something that was reasonable and that I could reach. I targeted 185 as what I needed to weigh. Then I kept that food diary you suggested, lowered my carbohydrates, and started an exercise routine. Nothing overboard or excessive. Just gradual. You know, a little at a time. I remember when you told me it would take six months, and I didn't want to believe it. I wanted something quick, something fast. I guess that's what we all want."

He was right. I remembered that conversation and his request for some "diet pills" to help get things started. I had reminded him of his blood pressure and that without significant and permanent lifestyle changes, most of us will fail at weight loss or quickly regain whatever we are able to initially lose.

"Anyway, that's why I wanted to thank you—for helping me lose that weight. That's the *how.* Now I want to tell you about the *why.*"

Jerry had plenty of reasons to want and need to lose weight. I closed his chart, sat back in the chair, and waited.

"We've got a pretty competitive bunch of people at work—probably why our company is so successful. Always looking for something to challenge each other with. Well, someone came up with the idea of a weight-loss competition. There's a group of us—about 12—who could all stand to lose a little or a lot of weight. We saw this as a kind of motivation, something that would be fun and good for us at the same time. We had to figure out the fairest way to do it, and decided that the person with the greatest percentage of weight lost would win the pot. Nothing big, just $20 apiece. But the winner would get $240 and bragging rights. The bragging part was the important thing.

"That was about when you advised me for the umpteenth time to lose some weight and told me again how to do it. Our group had decided the only thing off-limits was taking any weight-loss medication, either prescription or some of that over-the-counter stuff or what you can buy over the Internet. Anything else would be fair game.

"So I got organized, and you'd be proud of me. The first thing I did was go out and buy a notebook. I started keeping a food diary, and boy was it eye-opening. That probably helped as much as anything. It was hard at first—being honest with myself and writing down everything I ate. But then it became a kind of friend, and before I ate something, I found myself asking if I really wanted to write that down later. I passed on a lot of stuff—stuff I didn't need to be eating."

Jerry paused and shook his head. "I've got to admit though, those pounds didn't suddenly start melting away. I set a goal based on what you had told me—somewhere between 5 and 7 percent of my starting weight. I thought that would be reasonable, but what *wasn't* reasonable was my expectation that it would happen in a couple of weeks. I drank a ton of water, increased my exercising, and stopped eating all the white stuff— sugar, rice, potatoes, bread, and even pasta. The first week I lost about two pounds, which I was pretty happy with—until our group had its first weigh-in a week later. Some of those guys had dropped almost twice that amount and were making fun of me. I don't know how they did it, but they were already counting their money. And I was pretty discouraged.

"But I kept at it. I didn't do anything crazy, like running 20 miles a day or fasting for 48 hours. I just kept at it—slow and steady."

"The tortoise and the hare," I said.

"That's right. I was being slow and steady, like the tortoise. And I told myself that if I didn't win the pool, I'd still be a winner if I lost weight and was able to keep it off.

"After a couple of months, things began to change. I was still losing weight, but the other guys in my group weren't. In fact, most of them had regained the weight they had lost. It was usually the same excuse— 'Too hard to keep at it,' or 'This isn't worth the effort.' Two or three guys stayed with it, but they couldn't hang with me. Slow and steady, and at six months, I was the winner. I lost a little more than 7 percent of my initial weight, and I feel great. And I think I can keep it off, Doc. I'm not doing anything now that I can't keep doing for the rest of my life."

This was a great story and outcome, and I congratulated Jerry for what he had accomplished.

He was beaming again. He reached into his shirt pocket and took out a folded envelope.

"Here, Doc, I want you to have this. It's my winnings from the weight-loss competition."

I held up my hands and shook my head. "Jerry, you know I'm not going—"

"I knew you wouldn't accept anything like that." He stepped forward, grabbed my hand, and slapped the envelope into my palm. "This is a check made out to Camp Joy, the special-needs camp you and Barbara help with each summer. It'd mean a lot to me to be a part of that. You helped me win that weight-loss contest, and this is the least I can do."

I looked down at the envelope in my hand.

"And remember, Doc, it's the tortoise and the hare."

The wall. I had finally hit it. I reached the plateau I warned you about. Three weeks and nothing. Not an ounce. Nothing's changed—not what I'm eating or the water I'm drinking or my exercise routine. Yet I'm stuck. I've started keeping the diary again, and I'm going to have to find 100 calories a day. That would give me another pound in a month. But…where?

48

Eating Disorders, Part 1

Things You Need to Know

We now know a lot about eating disorders, but that hasn't always been the case. Just a few decades ago, the terms *anorexia* and *bulimia* were whispered, misunderstood, and considered to be the afflictions of movie stars and highly paid models. In medical circles, these real and dangerous problems were poorly understood and not considered worthy of serious attention—much less serious treatment.

That's all changed, and we have a much greater appreciation for the health hazards of these potentially devastating disorders and for their widespread prevalence. They affect millions of us—of every race, age, gender, size, locale, and educational level. Millions.

But what are we talking about here? What exactly is an eating disorder?

The *DSM-5* (the American Psychiatric Association's *Diagnostic and Statistical Manual of Mental Disorders*, fifth edition) characterizes these as a "persistent disturbance of eating that impairs health or psychological functioning." The *DSM-5* further separates these into specific categories based on established clinical findings and consistently observed symptoms. We're familiar with most of them—anorexia nervosa, bulimia nervosa, avoidant/restrictive food intake disorder, and binge eating disorder. These are the most common and potentially the most dangerous. We'll need to consider each of these separately.

But are you familiar with pica? Here's how the *DSM-5* describes this unusual behavior.

- Repeated eating of nonfood substances for at least one month, including cloth, dirt, chalk, paint, paper, coal, string, wool, gum, soap, and starch.

- This disorder is not appropriate for the individual's development level and is not culturally or socially accepted as being normal.

- Pica is not considered to be a suicidal behavior, such as the swallowing of harmful objects such as broken glass, nails, batteries, etc.

We don't know much about this problem, including its prevalence or even its long-term outcomes. But it's common enough for me to have seen a couple of cases during my training. One involved a young woman who came into the ER with a box of Argo cornstarch, munching on it during her visit for a sprained ankle. She was pregnant, severely anemic, and severely deficient in several vitamins. The other was a teenage boy who ate ice all day long. Not the kind of occasional crunching that aggravates your significant other, but the constant chewing of ice to the exclusion of any significant food intake. When he came to the ER, he was severely emaciated, painfully weak, and carrying a large cup of crushed ice.

That's hard to imagine, but it's true. As is the improbable rumination disorder. This is exactly what you might think it is, and for this diagnosis the *DSM-5* requires that each of the following symptoms persist for at least one month:

- Repeated regurgitation of food, which may be reswallowed, rechewed, or spit out.

- Regurgitation of food that is not due to an established medical condition (reflux disease/GERD).

- And regurgitation that does not occur as a part of other eating disorders, such as anorexia nervosa or binge eating.

I've never seen a case of this, at least one that I've recognized. But even though we don't know much about this eating disorder—such as how many of us have it and what's the outcome—it's real, and it's out there.

So assuming we'd be aware of the obvious presence of pica or the rumination disorder, what are the chances of us having one of the more common eating disorders? Or in the case of a friend or loved one, how can we help them identify this problem?

If you're reading this book to help lose weight because of a health condition (diabetes, high blood pressure, heart disease), or if you want to lose that last ten pounds in order to feel better, that's great and completely normal. That's why I've put this information together. But we have to face the reality that many aspects of our culture are obsessed with weight loss—and it begins at an early age. It's an obsession because it's unhealthy and in many ways unattainable. We mentioned movie stars and models earlier. If our goal is to look like them, we're not going to get there. And for many of us, including our teenagers, that can lead to some real problems with self-esteem and self-image. This is important stuff, and the obsession that leads to eating disorders is all too common.

Think you or a loved one might be at risk? How do we go about finding out? Fortunately a couple of simple screening instruments are effective in pointing us in the right direction. The first is called the SCOFF (Sick, Control, One stone, Fat, Food). Two or more positive responses indicate the potential diagnosis of an eating disorder. Try it.

- Do you make yourself sick (induce vomiting) because you feel uncomfortably full?

- Do you worry you have lost control over how much you eat?

- Have you recently lost more than one stone in a three-month period? (The developers of this survey are British, where weight is commonly expressed in stones—about 14 pounds. I guess they couldn't come up with another O.)

- Do you believe yourself to be fat when others say you are too thin?

- Would you say that food dominates your life?

Remember, two out of five of these puts us at risk. That holds true for another simple screening tool, the Eating Disorder Screen for Primary Care. Try this one too.

- Are you satisfied with your eating patterns? (No is the wrong answer.)

- Do you ever eat in secret? (Yes is obviously the wrong answer.)

- Does your weight affect the way you feel about yourself? (Yes is wrong.)

- Have any members of your family suffered with an eating disorder? (Yes is the wrong answer and puts us at risk.)

- Do you currently suffer with or have you ever suffered in the past with an eating disorder? (Yes is the wrong answer.)

Once again, two out of five wrong answers puts us at risk. If we fall into that category, we need to seek professional help.

One last screening tool is a little more involved and utilizes a 26-item questionnaire—the Eating Attitudes Test (EAT). This can be found online at www.eat-26.com. This is a great website and easy to use. You can request an analysis of your results, or you can use the cutoff point of 20 positive responses as indicating the increased risk for an eating disorder.

If you think you're at risk for one of these problems, get some help and get it now.

So that's how we can screen for this. Next we need to have a good understanding of the common eating disorders and how they can affect our health—and our lives.

49

Eating Disorders, Part 2

Binge Eating

Which do you think is the most common eating disorder in the United States? No fair peeking at the title of this chapter. If you knew it was binge eating, I'm proud of you. I didn't know it and was surprised to see the statistics.

Binge eating is in fact the most common, affecting somewhere between 2 and 3 percent of us, and slightly more women than men. To put that number into a little perspective, consider this: At a sold-out Ohio State University home football game, that 3 percent would represent more than 3100 of those people in the stadium. An even more impressive number is that many experts tell us that 30 to 40 percent of people seeking help for weight loss can be diagnosed with this disorder. So this is a common problem and a serious one.

This condition was first described in 1959 and was initially called the "night eating disorder." Its recognition as a real disease has been gradual. In fact, it was not designated as a distinct diagnosis until the late 1900s. Now it has its own code in the *Diagnostic and Statistical Manual of Mental Disorders*, fifth edition (*DSM-5*). And why might this be important? Two reasons. First, binge eating is now a clearly recognized, defined, and treatable disorder. And second, since it has its own diagnostic code, it should be recognized by most insurance companies and covered the same as other eating disorders and illnesses.

The name "binge eating" is descriptive of the problem, but we need to know the symptoms and requirements for its diagnosis. Here's what the *DSM-5* lists as the diagnostic criteria:

1. Recurrent episodes of binge eating. An episode is characterized by *both* of the following:

    a. Eating in a discrete period of time (within any two-hour period) an amount of food that is definitely larger than what most people would eat in a similar period of time under the same circumstances.

    b. The individual experiences a sense of lack of control over eating during the episode (feeling that one cannot stop eating or control what or how much one is eating).

2. The binge eating episodes are associated with *three or more* of the following:

    a. Eating much more rapidly than normal.

    b. Eating until feeling uncomfortably full.

    c. Eating large amounts of food when not feeling physically hungry.

    d. Eating alone because of feeling embarrassed by how much one is eating.

    e. Feeling disgusted with oneself, depressed, or very guilty afterward.

3. Marked distress regarding binge eating is present.

4. The binge eating occurs, on average, at least once a week for *three months.*

5. The binge eating is not associated with the recurrent use of inappropriate compensatory behaviors (purging) as in bulimia nervosa and does not occur exclusively during the course of bulimia nervosa or anorexia nervosa. In other words, the other eating disorders might involve occasional binge eating, but true binge eating must occur at times by itself.

So those are the things that need to be present in order to diagnose binge eating. Now we need to consider how this disorder can harm us.

First of all, binge eating is strongly associated with feelings of guilt, shame, anxiety, and depression. It is rare to have this disorder without experiencing some or all of these psychological effects. Untreated, this can lead to worsening of the eating disorder, estrangement from family and friends, and an increased risk for suicide.

The physical effects are significant as well. While as many as one-third of sufferers are of normal weight, the other two-thirds are obese and are at risk for those diseases that afflict people with elevated BMIs, such as heart disease, high blood pressure, diabetes, joint pain, high cholesterol levels, and sleep problems.

Think you or a loved one, friend, or family member might be at risk for having this eating disorder? It's important to remember that binge eating is an *expressive disorder*, meaning one that is an expression of deeper psychological problems. As such, we can look for clues that might tune us in to its possible presence. Here are some behaviors to keep in mind:

- Secretive food activities, such as eating in private (alone in the car), hiding food wrappers, or stealing or hoarding food.

- The disappearance of large amounts of food in short periods of time or lots of empty food containers or wrappers.

- Eating throughout the day with no planned mealtimes, engaging in periodic fasting or frequent dieting, and regularly skipping meals.

- Unusual behaviors while eating, such as not letting foods touch each other on the dinner plate.

- Frequently demonstrating feelings of anxiety, anger, shame, and worthlessness.

- Avoiding conflict and always trying to keep the peace.

- Difficulty expressing feelings and emotions.

- Demonstrating a strong need to be in control.

- Using that control to create opportunities for binge sessions.

As you can see, there are things here that are common to most of us, and by themselves don't constitute a significant threat to our physical and emotional well-being. But when we see many of these factors coming together, we need to consider the possibility of this eating disorder.

A couple of things to keep in mind: Not all binge eating is pathologic. Every one of us has overeaten at one time or another. That's not what we're talking about here. And not all of us with the binge-eating disorder are going to be overweight—only two-thirds. But the emotional and physical effects apply to everyone with this diagnosis. This is a real disease, and one that needs to be diagnosed and treated.

For more information about the binge eating disorder, a great resource is the National Eating Disorders Association (NEDA). Visit their website at www.nationaleatingdisorders.org.

50

Eating Disorders, Part 3

Bulimia Nervosa

The word *bulimia* comes from the Greek word meaning "ravenous hunger," and *nervosa* obviously refers to the nervous/emotional system. So understanding the root words should give us a good idea of what this disease might be about. And it does.

Bulimia is an eating disorder characterized by binge eating followed by an abnormal emotional response resulting in purging. It's important to understand this term *purging* and that it doesn't refer just to self-induced vomiting. Other efforts to lose weight might be taking laxatives, self-medicating with your own or someone else's diuretic (fluid pills), fasting, over-the-counter or prescription stimulants, and even excessive exercising.

The important point, and the one that sets bulimia apart from other eating disorders, is the purging after the binge eating. And just like the binge eating we discussed in the previous chapter, bulimia has its own diagnostic criteria and code and its own set of problems and complications. Let's consider those, starting with the physical effects of this disorder.

Commonly encountered physical signs include low blood pressure, a rapid heartbeat, dry skin, and problems associated with electrolyte abnormalities, such as low potassium or chloride. These electrolyte problems stem from the excessive vomiting frequently encountered with bulimia. Vomiting is also the cause of dental problems, including enamel erosion due to the acidity of regurgitated stomach contents and gum diseases.

Another telltale physical marker of this disease is calluses or scars on the backs of fingers due to the repeated trauma to these areas from front teeth during attempts at self-induced vomiting.

Frequent vomiting can also lead to inflammation of the esophagus, bleeding from the stomach or esophagus, menstrual irregularities and infertility in young women, and significant gastroesophageal reflux disease (GERD).

From an emotional standpoint—the *nervosa* component—we see low self-esteem, anxiety, depression, an increased incidence of substance abuse, and a higher risk of suicide and self-harm.

This is a serious condition, but how common is it? Not as common as binge eating, which we now know is the most frequently occurring eating disorder. But bulimia is not far behind. It affects as many as 1 to 2 percent of us, with experts in this area telling us this happens much more commonly among women, some placing the ratio of women to men as high as 9:1.

And this is tough to diagnose. Most of us with an eating disorder are reluctant to talk about it, and some of us are even unaware that this is a significant issue. Compounding that is the fact that most individuals with bulimia are of normal weight. This is different from what we saw with binge eating, and from what we will learn about anorexia nervosa.

So how do we make the diagnosis? Let's start with the basic features of this eating disorder. The diagnostic criteria cited by the *DSM-5* are:

- Repetitive episodes of binge eating. These must be discrete episodes of overeating during which the individual feels out of control with their excessive food consumption.

- These episodes are followed by "compensatory behaviors" in an effort to keep from gaining weight. These are the "purging" activities noted above.

- The diagnosis requires that this cycle of binging/purging happens at a minimum of once per week for a period of three months.

There is some overlap among all the eating disorders, making it even more difficult at times to establish the correct diagnosis. But it's important to do, and it can be done. As a physician, it's critical for me to be aware of this problem and to diligently pursue an accurate dietary and behavioral history. But this is where we as healthcare providers need help. Family members and loved ones frequently have a sense that something's going on, yet many times they're reluctant to mention it. They shouldn't be. Sometimes a life hangs in the balance.

What do we need to be looking for? Here's a list of things that should make your antennae stand on end:

- frequent self-weighing

- obsessive calorie counting

- ritualistic eating behaviors, such as cutting food into extremely small pieces

- binge eating behavior

- frequent trips to the bathroom after a meal

- a preoccupation with body image and weight

- misuse of over-the-counter laxatives and stimulants

- characteristic physical changes, such as dental problems, dry skin, and calluses on the backs of fingers

And remember, individuals with bulimia nervosa are frequently of a normal size and weight. So a serious and life-threatening eating disorder can occur in the absence of obesity or excessive weight loss. Just be aware, and don't be afraid to bring up the subject. A helpful tool we previously discussed is the SCOFF assessment (see chapter 48). It's a starting point.

The good news is that bulimia can be successfully treated and its health effects reversed. But it takes a team—concerned parents and loved ones, and experts in counseling and in treating this eating disorder.

Help is available.

51

Eating Disorders, Part 4

Anorexia Nervosa

Of the eating disorders, this is the most deadly. It literally results in starvation and all the medical complications associated with it. This one is not hard to detect, and we've all seen pictures of extreme cases. We may have friends or loved ones who have purposefully lost weight to an excessive degree and continue to do so. And while it may appear obvious to an observer, the involved person usually has no insight into what's happening to their body. There is a desire for thinness and an aversion to any body fat—sometimes to the point of death.

We've known about this disorder for hundreds of years, but the name *anorexia*, which means "no appetite," is a misnomer. Individuals with this disorder have not *lost* their appetite. They suppress it in order to lose weight and attain what they believe is the desirable body image.

The clinical features of anorexia nervosa are straightforward, including:

- persistent restriction of energy intake (food) that leads to an abnormally low body weight
- an intense fear of gaining weight or becoming fat, or persistent behavior that prevents weight gain
- a distorted perception of body weight and shape

Let's first consider the abnormally low body weight. This describes the severity of this order and is based on the BMI. Here is how the *Diagnostic and Statistical Manual of Mental Disorders (DSM-5)* classifies this:

- Mild: a BMI of 17 to 18.5
- Moderate: a BMI of 16 to 16.99
- Severe: a BMI of 15 to 15.99
- Extreme: a BMI less than 15

Here are a couple of examples:

- A teenage girl who is five feet six inches tall and weighs 102 pounds would be in the moderate category.
- The same girl weighing less than 90 pounds would be in the extreme category.

It turns out that there are two distinct subtypes of anorexia. The end result is the same—starvation. But how an individual gets there is different. And the treatment for a particular subtype will be different. Here's how these are defined.

Binge eating/purging type. These individuals utilize binge eating or display purging behavior as a means for losing weight. This is different from bulimia in that a person with anorexia does not maintain a healthy or normal weight but is significantly underweight. Those with bulimia nervosa are usually of normal weight—sometimes overweight.

Restricting type. This is just what it sounds like. These individuals restrict their intake of food, use diet pills, fast, and excessively exercise in order to lose weight. Some will exercise to keep weight off or prevent weight gain, while others eat only enough to barely stay alive.

Since the ultimate outcome is a picture of starvation, what are some of the physical changes that we see taking place?

Let's start with what happens when the human organism is starved. The process begins with the breakdown of protein and fat, all in an effort to maintain critical energy levels and cellular activities. As a result, cells start to shrink, and we see atrophy of the heart, brain, liver, intestines, and muscles. The severity of this depends upon the length and magnitude of the starvation.

Cardiovascular complications include a reduced cardiac muscle mass, fibrosis or scarring of the muscle, and heart valve problems. The smaller size of the heart can lead to dangerously low blood pressures and increasing fatigue. Patients with anorexia may complain of chest pain and heart palpitations. The electrical conduction system of the heart is also affected, and a slow heart rate can develop. Some reports indicate this can be profound and ultimately deadly, with pulse rates noted in the twenties. This slow heart rate manifests itself with weakness, fatigue, and light-headedness.

Absence of menstrual periods and infertility are well-documented problems, as is the development of osteoporosis.

If self-induced vomiting is a part of this picture, we can see all of the gastrointestinal complications we considered in our discussion of bulimia. In addition, drastically reduced food intake can lead to delayed emptying of the stomach and constipation.

The pulmonary system is also involved, with weakness and wasting of the muscles of respiration. Lack of adequate ventilation can lead to pneumonia and the complications that arise from aspiration.

The starvation of anorexia affects our bone marrow, and can result in dangerous anemias, low white-cell counts that can lead to overwhelming infections, and low platelet counts (easy bruising and uncontrolled bleeding).

Importantly, we now know that anorexia nervosa can lead to brain atrophy, with significant reductions in both gray and white matter.

Do these things go away with treatment? Sometimes, but not always. Once again, it depends on the length of time and severity of the starvation process. Some changes last a lifetime, thus affirming the need for a rapid diagnosis and effective treatment plan.

What are some of the tips to diagnosing this eating order?

Some skin changes should raise a few red flags. Yellowing of the skin is frequently present, as is dryness and scaling. Hair loss can occur, as well as evidence of the easy bruising noted above. Darkening of an area of skin (hyperpigmentation) can be seen, as well as a persistent itching. Slowly healing wounds are also part of the problem due to poor nutrition and an impairment of the immune/healing process. Something called *lanugo* should always raise the suspicion of this disorder. This is the development of fine, dark, downy hair on the trunk and face. In the setting of unexplained weight loss, this is an important warning sign.

There are a host of behavioral and psychological findings we need to be aware of:

- restlessness or hyperactivity
- concerns about eating in public
- a relentless and unfounded pursuit of thinness
- a fear of certain foods
- poor sleep
- inhibited expression of emotions
- a need to control one's environment
- inflexible thinking
- a lack of insight into the existence of a potential eating problem
- anxiety or depression
- an intentional resistance to treatment and weight gain
- an obsessive preoccupation with food manifested in unusual ways, such as hoarding and collecting recipes
- constantly counting calories
- consistently overestimating the number of calories in food
- overusing condiments and artificial sweeteners
- food-related rituals, including cutting food into small pieces, avoiding certain colors of food, and keeping food separate on the dinner plate

Some of these, occurring by themselves, are not pathologic. But if consistent, worsening, and combined with the weight loss we've discussed, they point to a more significant problem. Remember, this is the most deadly of the eating disorders and must be identified and treated.

But where do we turn? Your family physician is a good place to start.

And once again, I'd recommend the National Eating Disorders Association (NEDA) as a good source of accurate and helpful information (www.nationaleatingdisorders.org).

If at all suspicious of this disorder in a loved one, a friend, or even yourself, the most important thing to do is *act*.

52

Getting It Wrong

George Winters

"Mr. Winters seems a little anxious today," his nurse told me. "Heart rate is a little high and so is his blood pressure, but he says he was in a lot of traffic before getting here. Otherwise, everything's fine. I'll go check and see if his labs are back yet."

George Winters was a 42-year-old who had been coming to our office for more than a decade. He had always enjoyed good health, other than a slightly elevated blood pressure. But we had worked on that and gotten it under control.

I flipped open his chart and looked for the reason for today's visit. He had been in the office a couple of weeks earlier with what turned out to be a bad case of the flu, and he wasn't due for his annual exam for another six or seven months.

"Insurance exam."

That was an odd reason for coming to the office. Two or three years ago, we had completed a lengthy examination for a million-dollar life insurance policy for him. That shouldn't be changing now.

I closed the chart and walked down the hallway to his room.

"Good morning, George. Tell me how you're doing and about this insurance exam business."

Our eyes met and I was startled by his appearance.

Glassy-eyed and hollow-cheeked, he slumped on the exam table, leaning heavily against the wall behind him. One leg rocked listlessly back and forth.

"Hey, Robert. Just came by for a quick exam and to get some paperwork filled out."

How could he have changed so much in three weeks? What malignant process had I missed that was destroying his body? I pulled over the rolling stool, sat down, and stared at him.

"Yeah, I just need some basic stuff—you know, blood pressure, height, weight. My pressure should be good since we got started on that medication and cut out the salt."

He tried to chuckle, but what emerged from his throat was part cough, part croak. Something was very wrong. I glanced again at his chart. Blood pressure 100/60, heart rate 102, temperature 99.8, weight—he had lost 11 pounds in just over 21 days.

"What's the matter?" George was studying my face as I looked through his record. "Something's bothering you."

"Tell me about this insurance exam, George. Exactly what is that about?"

He shook his head and sighed. "Well, it's not really insurance—like life insurance or something. We did all that a couple of years ago, and that's all fine. This is something we do where I work. You know about all this health insurance stuff and all the changes that're taking place. Just like a lot of people, we've had to change policies a couple of times. And now in order to not have sky-high premiums, we have to do a health assessment. You get dinged if you smoke, and I get that. And if your blood pressure's high or you have diabetes that's not being treated, you get dinged for those too. I'm fine with all that, but the thing that's going to get me is my weight. According to my height, I shouldn't weigh more than 190 pounds. If I weigh more than that by the end of this month, I'll have to pay an extra $125 a month for my health insurance."

He wasn't at 190 yet. Though he had lost 11 pounds, he still weighed 196.

I told him what our nurse had written in his chart, and George shook his head. "I've only got a little more than a week."

His right hand was trembling—just a little. I hadn't noticed that this morning. This was something new.

"How have you managed to lose almost a dozen pounds since the last time you were here? That's a lot. You're not doing anything crazy, are you?"

I was half-joking, but when he flushed and looked away, I tensed.

"No, just cutting way down on what I eat and trying to exercise more. Cut out the sodas too—just like you told me."

His hand started to twitch now. George looked down and moved it behind him, hiding it from my sight.

A ton of red flags were popping up. Something was wrong, and I needed to find out.

"Let's take a look at you and make sure everything's okay."

His eyes were fine, with the pupils equal and quickly responding to my flashlight. I asked him to open his mouth. When he did, his tongue protruded and quivered uncontrollably. I was close enough to him now to notice the sweat dripping down his neck and disappearing underneath his shirt collar. More red flags.

His heart rate was fast—over 110—but regular. And when I checked the reflexes at his knees, he jerked and almost fell off the exam table.

"Whoa, take it easy, Doc."

I stepped back and studied the conundrum before me.

"George, are you taking any diet pills? Something you got off the Internet or somewhere?" Amphetamines and related drugs could cause these symptoms and were readily available if you knew where to look or who to ask.

"Nope, nothing like that."

He wouldn't look me in the eye, and I persisted.

"It's hard to lose that amount of weight in so short a time without taking something. Not unless you're on some kind of starvation diet—bread and water. And not much bread. If you're taking something, George, it's doing a number on you, and I need to know. You've got a tremor now, and your heart rate is fast. Your reflexes are way too active, you're sweating, and…"

The answer was right in front of me, and finally I understood. But how? Where did he get it?

George sighed loudly, stood up, and reached deep into his front pants pocket. He took out a medicine bottle and handed it to me.

The label was worn, but I could make out his wife's name, Amanda. And I could read the name of the medication—levothyroxine, 200 mcg. Her thyroid medicine—a healthy dose. This explained all of his symptoms and his rapid weight loss. He had induced his own hyperthyroidism, his own "thyroid storm"—dangerous and potentially deadly.

I looked at him and waited for an explanation, or at least a confession.

"I know, Doc. It's stupid. At first I felt fine, and the weight just seemed to drop off me. But then this started…" He held out his trembling hand. "And things just got worse. But that darned health assessment—$125 is a lot of money, and I…"

He fell silent and slowly got back on the exam table.

"George, let's talk about this."

53

A Little Weight-Loss Potpourri

Here's some hot-off-the-press information from several reputable medical journals. Future research may affirm or refute these points, but they're interesting—and make some sense. You might be able to put some of these to good use.

Education. The first item is probably too late for most of us. A study followed a group of more than 14,000 young people for more than 12 years. Among the things the researchers were interested in was the problem of weight gain and its timing with regard to college graduation and marriage. Previous information indicates that a college education is generally associated with a lower incidence of obesity. What these researchers discovered was that if a couple marries before graduating from college, they are 65 percent more likely to become obese than those who get married after college. While most of us gain weight after marriage, it seems that those who have graduated from college may have better coping and problem-solving skills than undergraduates, giving this group a better chance of avoiding excessive weight gain. Interesting, but too late for my wife and me.

Snacks. How about a snack? Feel a little guilty when you open the cabinet door and poke around? You might not have to. In fact, careful and creative snacking is an important part of losing weight and keeping it off. And it doesn't have to be difficult. Eating a protein-rich snack can reduce our appetites for much of the day and lessen the temptation to eat something less healthy or calorie laden.

But what's a healthy snack? We know that proteins are more slowly digested than carbohydrates and stick around in our systems for longer periods of time. Examples of these kinds of snacks are peanuts, almonds, limited cheese intake, and natural types of beef jerky (you have to be careful of added sugar). A study in the *Journal of Nutrition* found that teenagers who ate soy-based snacks (chocolate- or peanut-flavored soy pudding) consumed less sugar and fat during the day, felt less hungry, and consumed more protein in general. They also had improvements in some of their mood and cognitive functions. If you can improve the mood of a teenager, you've done something.

Another report stresses the finding that dietary protein is the most satiating of our major food groups: carbohydrates, fats, and proteins. With this in mind, they gave study participants a high-protein/low-carbohydrate breakfast drink each morning for several weeks. In addition to weight loss, these individuals reported less hunger during the day, reduced food consumption, and lower blood-sugar levels. These are all good things and easily achieved by paying attention to our choice of snacks. Reach for the protein.

Parents. Here's some sobering news for those of us with children. According to a large and ongoing study, parents aren't very good judges when it comes to whether or not their children are overweight. With parents of obese young boys, 97 percent thought their children were of normal weight. The parents of young girls did a little better, yet 88 percent of these parents perceived their obese children to be a normal size. How does this happen? And is it important?

First, it's important since childhood obesity is rapidly increasing in this country and around the world. If we as parents don't recognize the problem early, it becomes increasingly more difficult to manage. And how does this happen? Some experts attribute this to a lack of familiarity with and understanding of scientifically based growth charts. Instead, we compare our children's weights with those of their peers. If all of Johnny's friends are overweight, he must be doing okay.

And here's something else to be concerned about. Swedish researchers tell us that if a woman is overweight before or during pregnancy, her children are at an increased risk of developing type 1 diabetes. That's the kind that usually requires a lifetime of insulin therapy. But how much is the risk? It can be as much as a 33 percent increase. That's a lot, and something we need to keep in mind. And it's a lot of responsibility for those of us planning on having a family.

A supplement. Now for some good news. If you're looking for a magic pill to help you lose weight…well, you'll need to keep looking. But there is something that might help, and it *does* come in the form of a pill. This is a safe and familiar supplement, something that's been getting a lot of attention lately in the press and in medical circles—vitamin D. That's right, good old vitamin D. We know it does a lot of good things for us, but if we all had our levels checked, most of us would be deficient. It turns out that the amount of sunshine you get each day doesn't have a significant impact on the level of vitamin D in your blood. That's probably a good thing since the majority of us need to spend less time in the sun anyway. But if your level is low, it can easily be raised by a daily dose of vitamin D3—somewhere around 2000 to 3000 units. And if you happen to be overweight and your level is low and you fix it, several good things may happen. Along with paying attention to your calorie intake, vitamin D supplementation can result in weight loss and a reduction in waist circumference. Again, it's not a magic pill, but in conjunction with an overall weight-loss program, this needs to be a part of the battle plan.

Spice. And for those of us who think spicy foods are only for crazy Uncle Fred down in New Orleans, it may be time to get over it and get out the hot sauce. We've known for a long time that chili peppers can clear our sinuses and tear glands. Now we have breaking news that the main component of chili, capsaicin, can help induce weight loss—or at least prevent gaining some of those unwanted pounds. The mechanism of action seems plausible, since capsaicin can induce thermogenesis (the internal production of heat). The thought is that this action increases the burning of energy, thus consuming calories at a more rapid than normal rate. Granted, these initial studies have been performed only on mice, but hey, we've got to start somewhere.

So these are a few things that might help in your quest to control your weight and that of your children.

54

Doctor, It's Just Got to Be Glandular

In my experience, that statement is usually coming from a concerned mother regarding her overweight teenage daughter. But I also hear it from women and men who have struggled for years to lose weight without any meaningful success. They're trying to find a reasonable and simple explanation for this failure—hoping that there might be a quick fix. For the majority of us, though, there is no glandular cause of our obesity. It all comes back to that balance between what we take in and what we burn up.

However, there are a few of us who *can* blame our glands for our added pounds. The first such problem has to do with an underactive thyroid gland—hypothyroidism. This wouldn't be a likely diagnosis in the teenager mentioned above, but it does become a factor as we grow older—for men and for women. As many as 5 percent of Americans have some degree of an underactive thyroid, including Oprah Winfrey, Linda Ronstadt, Sofia Vergara, the late president John Adams, and Doxology, our golden retriever. It manifests itself with fatigue, cold intolerance, poor memory and concentration, and obesity, despite having a poor appetite. This should be something your physician routinely checks for, but it can slip up on us. When corrected, we'll feel much better, have more energy, and yes, lose some weight.

The other glandular cause of weight gain is more subtle, yet it's relatively common and is the most frequently occurring obesity-related endocrine syndrome in females—polycystic ovary syndrome (PCOS). Statistics vary, but a reasonable estimate is that as many as 1 in 40 women—almost seven million females—may have this condition, including Victoria Beckham, Emma Thompson, and Jillian Michaels. While we don't know what causes this syndrome, we do know what it looks like.

Symptoms frequently begin in adolescence and present as increased facial and body hair, moderate to severe acne (more than ten facial lesions at one time), abnormal menstrual cycles and infertility, and obesity. The name *polycystic* comes from the ultrasound findings of an increased number of cysts (more than 12 on one or both ovaries), although the presence of these cysts is not required to make the diagnosis.

The syndrome can also be associated with mood changes, including anxiety and depression, an impaired quality of life, and even with eating disorders, including binge eating.

We're concerned here with the issue of obesity in these young women with PCOS. Only about 50 percent of those with this diagnosis are obese, but when present, the obesity is difficult to manage and almost always "central" (the apple-shaped body image we discussed in an earlier chapter). Because of this central or visceral obesity, women with PCOS are at an increased risk for the development of heart disease, diabetes, and high blood pressure. That makes it important to establish an accurate diagnosis and begin treatment.

Fortunately, the mainstay of this treatment is a common and inexpensive medication, metformin. You might recognize this as one of the medicines used for the treatment of diabetes. Women with PCOS share some of the same problems as those with diabetes, including the development of significant insulin resistance. In addition to helping with this specific problem, metformin provides the added benefit of weight loss and maintenance. This is a very treatable condition, but first it has to be considered as a possibility and correctly diagnosed.

So, Momma, you might be right about your daughter's glandular problem. It should be something we take seriously.

55

Frequently Asked Questions

Each day, we help many of our patients with their weight-loss aspirations. We assist them with setting an appropriate goal, guide them with appropriate and proven lifestyle changes, and answer their many questions. By taking the time to listen and consider these questions, we've uncovered a lot of misinformation surrounding this important topic.

Q. A friend of mine went on the grapefruit diet for a couple of weeks and lost a lot of weight. How many grapefruits should I be eating each day, and is it okay to eat the pink ones?

Grapefruit—either the white or pink variety—is a good source of vitamin C, fiber, and lycopene, and it's low in calories. But the so-called grapefruit diet is not a diet or weight-loss plan. It falls squarely in the fad category and should be avoided.

Q. A fraternity brother of mine once told me that since the calories in alcohol were "empty," drinking beer and wine won't cause you to gain weight. Was he right?

First, I'd like to know his belt size and then whether he graduated. The empty calories in alcohol he refers to have to do with their lack of any nutritional value, not in their inability to induce weight gain. A calorie is a calorie is a calorie.

Q. I've always heard that a calorie of fat will make you gain more weight than a calorie of protein. How do carbohydrates compare?

Hmm. Didn't we just say that a calorie is a calorie is a calorie? You might be confusing this with the calories in one *gram* of fat, which would be nine, while one gram of protein and one gram of carbohydrate each contain four calories.

Q. My cousin bought some diet stuff over the Internet—May Wong, I think. He's lost some weight but says it makes him feel funny. I'd like to lose about 15 pounds and was wondering if this is something I should try.

This is an easy one. Your cousin is probably taking Ma Huang, and no wonder he feels funny. The active ingredient is ephedra, a chemical that can increase heart rate and blood pressure and cause dizziness. This has been banned by the FDA, and for good reason. Yet it can easily be found on the Internet under such names as Yellow Devils, Ripped Power, Green Stinger, and Yellow Bullet. The fine print of some of these ads should tell us all we need to know: "Taking more than the recommended amount can result in heart attack, stroke, seizure, and death."

Keep in mind that there is no recommended or safe amount. Stay away from this stuff. And tell your cousin.

Q. When my mother sent me to the grocery store for eggs and milk, she always told me to go straight to the back and not look at all the stuff on the shelves. I was always scared to look, and I've wondered if she was just spoofing me. What do you think?

I think your mother was a wise woman. Supermarkets have been in the food-selling business for a long time, and they've developed an art to go along with the science. The next time you're in a grocery store, notice where they place the staples—eggs, bread, milk. You'll find them in the back of the store, requiring you to pass by long and laden aisles of processed and glitzy food products. Beware. Processed foods are almost always loaded with bad stuff. And be aware of this and other sales techniques.

Q. A friend at work puts heavy cream in his coffee all the time. I told him he was crazy and was going to gain weight. He should be using nondairy creamer, right?

Sorry, but I must disagree. Your friend's heavy cream is causing him no harm since it contains only a few calories (depending on how much he uses) and no carbs. And as to which one of you is crazy, you need to read the label of your nondairy creamer.

Q. My home-economics teacher in high school used to always tell us to use spices when we cooked—that it would make our food taste better, keep us healthy, and help us lose weight. Now that I'm trying to drop a few pounds, I'm trying to remember those spices. Seems that most of them started with the letter C. Any idea, or was she wrong?

The latest and growing evidence says she was right. And she was probably referring to cardamom, cumin, and coriander, all of which have shown evidence of helping with weight loss in addition to being potent antioxidants. Oh, and don't forget curry, usually a combination of coriander, cumin, and turmeric. It's another antioxidant and is known to lower cholesterol levels and help you lose weight.

Q. My girlfriend called me a big dummy when I told her I've never heard of harissa. What gives here?

First, I'd venture that your girlfriend is rather trendy. Harissa is becoming somewhat of a stylish fad, with its origins found in Tunisia. It's a chili-pepper paste, usually composed of various chili peppers, spices, herbs, coriander or sesame seeds, and olive oil. It won't help you lose weight or clear your sinuses, but it'll make your eyes water. I can't speak to the big dummy part.

Q. I read somewhere that the BMI is not the best way to determine whether you're overweight. What do you think?

That's a good question and a tough one. Most experts agree that obesity can be defined as a body fat percentage of more than 25 percent in men and 35 percent in women. The problem comes when we try to measure that. A *direct* method would be underwater weighing (not something that's routinely done in our office) or bioelectrical impedance measurement (not all that accurate). The BMI is an *indirect* method of determining body composition and is prone to some potential errors. One of these might be inaccurate measurements of height and weight, and another would be that muscular individuals might be misclassified as being obese since muscle weighs more than fat. Yet for all its flaws, the BMI is the best and simplest method we currently have to guide us with this important issue.

Q. I know you're not supposed to eat rice and potatoes on the low-carb diet, but I was told brown rice and sweet potatoes were fine. I've been eating those, but I can't seem to lose weight. Any ideas?

You just answered your own question. No, they're not all right. Brown rice, dirty rice, wild rice—all the same when it comes to carbs. And they don't call it a "sweet" potato for nothing. The same is true for bread. Multigrain, healthy-grain, all-natural—check out the carbohydrate content on the label. This is where we need to understand the glycemic index of foods and put it to use. If you're trying to significantly reduce your carbohydrate intake, you'll need to avoid or at least reduce everything white—sugar, rice, potatoes, pasta, bread. All of our comfort foods. But that's the way it is. And regarding rice—one of my favorite comfort foods—I have had several of my diabetic patients tell me that rice does a real number on their blood sugars. More so than anything else.

Q. My girlfriend is trying to lose some weight and just seemed to stall out. The scales haven't budged in two or three weeks. She said something about hitting a plateau, but I told her she must be sneaking some extra food somewhere. That made her mad, but I know you'll agree with me.

I'll only agree that you'll probably soon be looking for a new girlfriend. She's right about this one. Most of us will reach a plateau when we're trying to lose weight. Nothing seems to help, and the scales are frozen—maybe even going up. It's a natural occurrence with our bodies slowing down our metabolism to prevent what it perceives as starvation. Natural, but frustrating.

It can be overcome with a little time and perseverance, and there are a couple of things we need to do. The first is to increase our physical activity—adding another 15 to 20 minutes a day. Then we need to increase our water intake—a total of at least six to eight eight-ounce glasses. And lastly, we need to check our food labels for hidden carbohydrates. Remember that low-fat salad dressings take out the fat and add a lot of sugar. Sneaky, but that happens in a lot of places. You have to be on the lookout. And good luck with your new girlfriend.

Q. I have a friend who's a personal trainer. She says the best time of day to exercise is early in the morning. But I thought that's when most heart attacks occur. What do you recommend?

You're right about the heart attacks. The early morning hours are the most dangerous from a cardiac standpoint, but not due to exercise. As long as you spend some time moving around and warming up before jumping right into your routine, you should be fine. In fact, some experts believe that aerobic exercise early in the morning is more effective for fat loss. It raises your metabolism for the rest of the day, and because you've been fasting overnight and used up your stores of energy, the body will use up more fat while you exercise. Makes sense, but you'll have to see how it works for you.

Q. The last time I was in the office, you recommended the low-carb diet for me. You said eating eggs would be okay, and I've been eating one or two every day. The other night I was talking with my second cousin's brother's girlfriend. She's a nutritionist and says you're out of your mind and that I should eat only one egg a month, and only on a Thursday when it's a full moon. What have you got to say about that?

Unfortunately, she's probably right about me being out of my mind, but not about eating eggs. Let's take a look at your chart. Hmm…over the last five weeks, you've lost eight pounds, your blood pressure is perfect, and your cholesterol and triglycerides are now normal. What have *you* got to say about *that*?

Q. Some of us at work have been trying out this new Paleo diet, and it seems to be helping. But my wife says it's just a fad and that before long, I'll be looking like a caveman. She says I've been acting like one for a long time, but is she right? I mean about the fad thing?

She might be right about all of it. The Paleolithic diet is another in a long line of diet variations searching for a niche. There are aspects of this that make sense, such as eating berries, nuts, and meat. But the meat needs to be lean, and the exclusion of dairy products, grains, and legumes is hard to swallow. We know what works for a healthy diet, and unless solid research leads us elsewhere, we don't need to spend our time and money chasing another newly pronounced "wonder diet."

56

When You Reach the Plateau

It will happen to all of us. We'll reach a point in our attempts to lose weight where it all stops. The numbers on the scale are frozen, and try as we might, we just can't get below that maddening set of digits. We've plateaued.

If it hasn't already happened to you, get ready—it will. There might be a slim minority of us who are able to zip to our weight-loss goal and are never faced with this frustration. But they are fortunate and few. I'm not one of them. I've been there. (Several times, I must admit.)

So it's likely to happen, and we need to be prepared to meet it head-on. You might be there right now and are unable to pierce that impregnable barrier and reach your weight-loss target. That might be why you're reading this book in the first place—to seek answers and help. There are answers, and there is help. Let's get organized and develop a battle plan.

We've mentioned before that one of the laws of nature turns out to be cruel, at least for those of us intentionally trying to lose weight. *Intentional* is the key word here, and *cruel* might be a little harsh, since this natural phenomenon is actually something designed to save our lives. As we lose weight, our bodies sense that something is happening, something we're wired to perceive as dangerous. We're eating less or burning more calories...in a sense, we're starving. In an effort of self-preservation, our metabolism is reset—the way we generate energy is changed. We shift gears, needing fewer calories to keep essential activities going, and our weight loss slows.

It happens to everyone. After all, it's a law of nature. We've been at a

certain weight for a while, and that has become our new normal. But that
set point can be readjusted, and our intentional weight loss can continue.
The resetting can take a few weeks or months, but as long as we're aware
of what's going on, we can anticipate it, not become frustrated, and not
give up.

That may be part of the reason for our plateau, but more than likely
other things are going on. These will be the factors we need to identify
and change. And we can.

The first step is to reassess our goal. No, don't skip down to the next
point. This is important. Remember that most of us will set a weight-loss
target that is unrealistic. The average is 30 percent of our current weight.
For me, that would be losing 60 pounds. Not going to happen, and I'll
have reached a plateau long before that mark, given up, and in frustration
probably gained a few pounds. (That's another law of nature.) A 5 to 7
percent goal within six months is reasonable, and for most of us, achievable. Set that mark, get there, and then reassess. If you still want or need
to lose more weight, set another goal, but be patient. And most importantly, be realistic.

Now we need to pull out our food diaries once more. Again, don't
skip to the next point. We've stressed how important this activity is for
a successful weight-loss effort. It's even more important if we're going to
get beyond our plateau. In addition to the points we made in chapter 11
about what we need to be keeping track of, here's what we need to be paying close attention to and to record—accurately and honestly:

Exercise. How much exercise are we getting? Not at work or through
some form of estimation, but how many minutes of leisure-time, moderate activity are we achieving each day? Record the activity and the specific
number of minutes. Our goal is 150 minutes a week of moderate exercise.
Look for a trend with this—maybe consistent days of the week where you
might be falling short. Once you have an accurate assessment of your average weekly exercise minutes, add some to your routine. Start with another
5 minutes a day. That gives you another 35 minutes every seven days, and
maybe as many as another 200 calories a week burned (more than 800
a month). This quickly adds up, and unless we're compensating by eating more, this will tip the balance of energy intake and energy expenditure in our favor.

Water. How much water are we drinking? The admonition of "six to eight glasses each day" is probably not enough. Record this amount, as well as other liquids you consume each day. Water is the best thing here, and it's the easiest and cheapest (assuming you're not buying the bottled stuff). Most of us aren't drinking enough and will need to increase our daily consumption by a quart or so. This will help, and I'm living proof. This is where I usually fall short and hit a plateau. When I'm working, I forget about drinking and don't get nearly enough water. It takes a conscious effort and plan, but adequate water intake is essential if we're going to lose weight. And staying hydrated helps everything else, including the way we feel.

That's your food diary, and if we're serious about moving beyond our plateau, we'll be serious about dusting off our notebook and putting it to use.

While we're doing these things, we need to closely evaluate what we're eating and be constantly vigilant for those killers of every weight-loss effort—the hidden carbs. Don't think this is important or has any real effect on our plateau? Well, we need to think again.

We've considered how carbohydrates can wreak havoc on our bodies through their stimulation of insulin release, and how this process leads to weight gain. Limiting carbohydrate intake is an essential part of every successful and sustainable weight-loss plan. But things seem to be stacked against us. Many of these carbs *are* hidden, and we find them in places we least suspect.

Here's a simple example—your favorite salad dressing. A healthy salad is an important part of every diet, but it's hard to eat that lettuce or spinach without something to add some flavor and moisture. Olive oil and balsamic vinegar is a good choice, but most of us have our preferred dressings. The trap set for us is the work of the food-processing industry. We are tempted to switch from our regular ranch dressing (just a few carbs per serving) to the "low calorie" or "healthy" choice. The label is the tip-off, and we have to look. The manufacturers of these dressings lower the fat content and replace it with a ton of sugar. Fewer calories, true, but now loaded with carbs. Check the labels, and you'll be surprised.

That's just one area where we encounter hidden carbs. There are many others, and a quick and informed inspection of nutrition labels will help ferret these out. It's important, and if you take a hard look at this, you'll be able to eliminate these unnecessary and hidden carbohydrates. Pretty soon, you won't need to read the labels. You'll just know, and you'll avoid these diet killers.

So if you've reached a plateau, try these things. Most of my patients, when they honestly and aggressively make these changes, are able to move beyond that impasse and lower the reading on their scales. You can too.

57

Ghrelin and Leptin

The Future of Weight Loss?

Ghrelin and leptin. Sounds like the names of long-forgotten characters from a Grimm's fairy tale. It turns out that we'll need to know something about these two hormones, especially as they pertain to weight loss, gain, and management. Though leptin was first described in 1994 and ghrelin seven years later, we are still just scratching the surface in our understanding of how these two chemicals impact the complex area of metabolic endocrinology.

Ghrelin

Pronounced "GREL-in," this substance is now widely known as the hunger hormone. It's produced in several areas of the gastrointestinal tract with most of this occurring in the stomach and duodenum. When the stomach is empty, specialized cells release ghrelin, which then travels through the bloodstream to the brain. There it stimulates receptors in the hypothalamus that produce sensations of hunger and the search for food. Once our stomach becomes distended after a meal, less ghrelin is produced, and we are no longer hungry. This sounds like a pretty simple loop, and if we could flip a couple of switches, we should be able to manipulate this hormone to our advantage.

Since ghrelin can cross directly from our bloodstream into our brain (something larger molecules and substances are not able to do), we should be able to manufacture it, inject it into our system, and predict the effects. This turns out to be the case. In animal studies and a few human experiments, injected ghrelin induces an increase in appetite and subsequent weight gain. This might turn out to be important for those of us who are unable to maintain a healthy body mass, including the weight loss associated with cancer. Research in this area is ongoing, and we'll have to wait and see how important this will ultimately be.

But since this is a book about weight loss, we want to flip the other switch, don't we? If we could block the action of ghrelin and prevent the natural hunger response produced by an empty stomach, we should be able to reduce our intake of food and lose weight. This is what happens when rodents and pigs are given "ghrelin blockers"—they lose weight. Unfortunately, no blockers are currently approved for use in humans. This is another of those wait-and-see areas of weight-loss management. And while this appears to be a simple hormonal loop, this whole area of research gets more complicated and intertwined in the face of exploding knowledge.

Exciting stuff, but we're not there yet. However, we do know a couple of things that we can put to good use. First, ghrelin levels (and the incidence of obesity itself) increase in those of us who don't get enough sleep. This is a straightforward relationship, with fewer hours of sleep resulting in increasing blood levels of ghrelin.

And there seems to be a connection between ghrelin levels and increased intake of fish oil (omega-3 fatty acids). It might have to do with some degree of natural blocking, but those of us with higher intake of these oils tend to be less hungry and better able to lose weight.

Ghrelin has some interesting positive effects as well. It's important in maintaining healthy blood vessels, and there is some indication that this hormone improves our ability to learn and remember. This is supported by some evidence that we learn better when our stomachs are empty.

The last piece of information to consider about ghrelin is that blood levels naturally increase as we grow older. That's just not fair, but it may help to explain why losing weight gets more and more difficult with each passing year.

Leptin

Now let's consider leptin. It's important to remember that when we talk about the discovery of anything that pertains to our bodies or our universe, we're not inventing anything new. We're simply unlocking some things that heretofore have remained a mystery. The interactions of leptin and its cousin ghrelin are among the mysteries that declare the wonderful intricacies of our bodies. Fearfully and wonderfully made indeed.

So we have leptin, a hormone chiefly produced in the fat cells scattered throughout our body. When our fat stores are plentiful—and whose aren't?—leptin is released and makes its way to our brain, where it acts in the same area that ghrelin exerts its effects. Leptin *suppresses* our appetite, thus reducing the amount of our food intake and modulating the fat stored in our fat cells. As proof of this, as our BMI and body fat increase, leptin production increases and blood levels rise. We're not as hungry. As further evidence of the importance of this hormone, a few of us have a significant leptin deficiency. Despite our best efforts, weight loss becomes almost impossible, and obesity is one of the hallmarks of this condition. Treatment with leptin can dramatically reduce food consumption and result in significant weight loss.

So why doesn't everyone who wants to lose weight just take some leptin every morning? That was the initial hope, but things haven't worked out that way. If you're leptin deficient (a rare condition), taking leptin will result in weight loss. But for the overwhelming majority of us, it won't help. I told you this was complex, and this is one of those twisty turns that we've uncovered. As with insulin, we can become leptin resistant, meaning that ever-increasing amounts of leptin have ever-diminishing effects. It stops working. That's why a lot of the initial excitement surrounding this hormone has waned. It might still prove to be useful, but at present, it remains the focus of ongoing research and not part of our weight-loss armamentarium.

Promising, but no magic bullet just yet.

58

A Little Perspective

Here are some things we need to keep in mind as we consider how to lose some weight.

At any given moment, more than two-thirds of all adults in the United States are either trying to lose weight or maintain it. Yet less than 20 percent of these people are actually eating fewer calories than they were before starting, nor are they getting 150 minutes of physical activity each week—both essentials for success.

Want to know what a little weight loss might feel like? Find something that weighs ten pounds (a barbell is ideal) and carry it around with you for a while—maybe for as little as 15 minutes. It doesn't take very long for that small amount to become heavy. Imagine that extra weight banging away at your knees and hips and back. Then put it down and feel the relief.

Three important markers of success include a weight loss of more than four and a half pounds in four weeks, regular attendance in some form of weight-loss program, and the belief that your weight can be controlled.

Here's a simple but effective trick to add to your weight-loss program. Try standing. Yes, standing. Those of us who spend at least one-fourth of our time standing each day have a significantly reduced chance of becoming obese. This simple activity can actually help us lose weight. When we combine that with the guidelines for leisure-time physical activity (150 minutes a week of moderate exercise), the odds get even better, as does our risk of developing the metabolic syndrome.

Here's a disturbing trend: From 2000 to 2012, American households doubled their purchases of food from convenience stores, warehouse clubs, and mass merchandisers, while food bought in grocery stores continued its downhill slide. Why disturbing? You don't find many fresh vegetables and fruit in convenience stores, and many of the items bought outside of grocery stores are packaged products that contain a lot of salt and sugar. Another part of the obesity epidemic.

Lest we take all of this and ourselves too seriously, consider some of these pearls of wisdom from an assortment of individuals about their own experiences with losing weight.

> "I've been on a diet for fourteen days, and all I've lost so far is two weeks."
>
> *Totie Fields*

> "I tried every diet in the book. I tried some that weren't in the book. I tried eating the book. It tasted better than most of the diets."
>
> *Dolly Parton*

> "The second day of a diet is always easier than the first. By the second day, you're off it."
>
> *Jackie Gleason*

> "A diet is the penalty we pay for exceeding the feed limit."
>
> *anonymous*

> "Probably nothing in the world arouses more false hopes than the first four hours of a diet."
>
> *Dan Bennett*

> "The cardiologist's diet: If it tastes good, spit it out."
>
> *anonymous*

"The biggest seller is cookbooks and the second is diet books—
how not to eat what you've just learned to cook."

Andy Rooney

"I've been on a constant diet for the last two decades. I've lost
a total of 789 pounds. By all accounts, I should be hanging
from a charm bracelet."

Erma Bombeck

"Most things in life are easy to lose and hard to gain. Not so
with our weight."

anonymous

"If only losing weight was as easy as losing my cell phone, my
keys, my temper, or even my mind, I'd be skinny."

anonymous

Just a little perspective.

59

Putting It All Together

If you're one of the 30 percent of us who are trying to lose some weight—no matter the reason—don't give up hope. It takes a plan, a big dose of discipline, and some help. You'll find a lot of that help in these pages—things that you'll need to know and do as you journey toward a successful weight-loss goal.

There's a lot of information here, and I've organized the key chapters that will guide you to specific topics.

1. First, we need to understand why achieving a desirable and healthy weight is important. Obesity leads to a lot of major problems, most of which can be avoided.

Chapter 2, "What's the Big Deal?"
Chapter 3, "Obesity and Heart Disease"
Chapter 4, "Obesity and the Development of Diabetes"
Chapter 5, "Obesity and Some Other Bad Stuff"
Chapter 6, "The Metabolic Syndrome"

2. Next, there are some things we'll need to understand as we embark on our weight-loss journey.

Chapter 12, "What's This Waist-Hip Ratio Business?:
     Comparing Apples to Pears"
Chapter 13, "The Lowly Calorie: Unloved, Unappreciated,
     Yet So Important"

Chapter 18, "Water, Water Everywhere..."
Chapter 27, "'He Created Them Male and Female'"
Chapter 56, "When You Reach the Plateau"
Chapter 57, "Ghrelin and Leptin"

3. Now we need to have a plan.
Chapter 8, "Setting a Goal"
Chapter 10, "Let's Get Started!"
Chapter 11, "Keeping a Food Journal"

4. As with most things, evaluation of our lifestyle is critically important, followed by making the appropriate and necessary changes.
Chapter 14, "Exercise: Ya Gotta Get Movin'"
Chapter 15, "Exercise: Overcoming the Yo-Yo"

5. Choosing what we need to eat is central to our weight-loss efforts. How do we make that decision?
Chapter 19, "What Am I Supposed to Be Eating?"
Chapter 20, "What Diet Choices Are There?"
Chapter 21, "The Fad Diets: They Come and Go"
Chapter 22, "Why Low-Fat Diets Don't Work"
Chapter 23, "The Low-Carbohydrate Approach"
Chapter 24, "The Low-Carb Diet: What It Looks Like"
Chapter 25, "What's the Best Diet?: One Clear Choice"
Chapter 26, "The Mediterranean Diet: What It Looks Like"

6. We're bombarded by ads for all kinds of weight-loss products and herbal concoctions. How do we make sense of all that?
Chapter 29, "Complementary and Alternative Medicine (CAM)"
Chapter 30, "CAM and Weight Loss: Dietary Supplements"

7. In order to achieve our weight-loss goal, many of us will need help in the form of medication.
Chapter 32, "Prescription Weight-Loss Medicines:
  Is One Right for Me?"
Chapter 33, "Prescription Weight-Loss Medicines:
  Drugs That Alter Fat Digestion"
Chapter 34, "Prescription Weight-Loss Medicines:
  Serotonin Activators"

Chapter 35, "Prescription Weight-Loss Medicines:
   The Stimulants"
Chapter 36, "Prescription Weight-Loss Medicines:
   The Combinations"

8. What are we to make of the commercial weight-loss plans? Can they help us?
Chapter 39, "Commercial Weight-Loss Plans: Do They Work and
   Are They Worth It?"
Chapter 40, "Jenny Craig"
Chapter 41, "Weight Watchers"
Chapter 42, "Nutrisystem"

*9. Some of us will need to lose more than ten pounds. It may be much more
than that if we are going to save our lives, and we'll need to consider bariat-
ric surgery.*
Chapter 43, "Bariatric Surgery: What Are We Talking About?"
Chapter 44, "Bariatric Surgery: What Are Our Choices?"
Chapter 45, "Bariatric Surgery: The Pros, the Cons, and
   What You Can Expect"
Chapter 46, "Choosing a Bariatric Surgeon:
   Does It Make a Difference?"

*10. Sometimes things can go wrong. We need to know what these are and how
to recognize them.*
Chapter 48, "Eating Disorders: Things You Need to Know"
Chapter 49, "Eating Disorders: Binge Eating"
Chapter 50, "Eating Disorders: Bulimia Nervosa"
Chapter 51, "Eating Disorders: Anorexia Nervosa"

11. And then for some fun stuff.
Chapter 7, "A Brief History of Weight Loss"
Chapter 53, "A Little Weight-Loss Potpourri"
Chapter 55, "Frequently Asked Questions"
Chapter 58, "A Little Perspective"

12. The key to making it happen.
Chapter 17, "Discipline: A Muscle in Need of Exercise"

A successful weight-loss effort is all about understanding our body, making a commitment, finding balance, and exercising our discipline muscle. You can do it. Just get started!

> I can do all this through [Christ] who gives me strength.
>
> *Philippians 4:13*

60

Dave Jernigan: Victory!

Dave was beaming and with good reason. He had reached his weight-loss goal.

It had been eight weeks since his last visit, and I had barely closed the exam room door when he exclaimed, "We did it! I guess you saw my chart. I'm at my 'fighting weight,' as you call it. And I feel great!"

"*You* did it, Dave. And congratulations."

I tossed his chart onto the exam table and stood in front him. He *had* done it—something that most of us never quite do. But he had been determined and disciplined.

"Doc, I took that medicine you gave me for about two months. It worked great, and it helped me control my appetite. The pounds started coming off, and pretty soon I reached the goal we set. I decided to stop the pills and see if I could keep the weight off. And you know what? I have. I feel great. And I want to stay this way. I know what to do, and I'm going to stick with it."

Somehow, I believed he would.

He was in the office six months later for a routine checkup. His blood pressure was perfect, his labs were good, and his weight…exactly the same.

Victory!

Some Final Thoughts

Whatever your weight-loss goal—whether it's ten pounds or even more—you can get there. It will take determination and discipline, with a laser-like focus on your diet and physical activity. But the results will be worth it, not only with how you feel but with your health and overall well-being.

I want to know how you do, so please share your thoughts and experiences with me at robertlesslie.com.

And good luck!

It's been a victory for me as well—almost. I've lost a total of nine pounds, knocking on the door of my ten-pound goal. I whipped the plateau by finding those 100 calories a day. It was simple, really. I drink about six cups of coffee a day, with a little cream. I looked at those extra calories and started drinking my coffee black. And that did it. Sometimes it doesn't take much. Now for that last pound...

About the Author

Bestselling author **Dr. Robert Lesslie** is a physician with more than 30 years of experience working in or directing fast-paced, intense ER environments. He is now the co-owner and medical director of two urgent-care facilities. He has written *60 Ways to Lower Your Blood Pressure, 60 Ways to Lower Your Cholesterol, Notes from a Doctor's Pocket, Angels on the Night Shift, Angels and Heroes, Angels on Call, Miracles in the ER*, and *Angels in the ER* (over 400,000 copies sold) as well as newspaper and magazine columns and human-interest stories. He and his wife, Barbara, live in South Carolina. Together they have raised four children—Lori, Amy, Robbie, and Jeffrey—and are now enjoying eight grandchildren.

More Great Harvest House
Books by Dr. Robert Lesslie

More help for enjoying a healthier and longer life…

60 Ways to Lower Your Cholesterol

60 Ways to Lower Your Blood Pressure

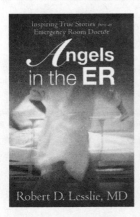
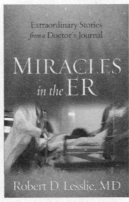
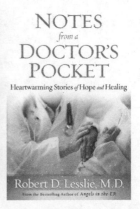

Heartwarming stories from Dr. Lesslie's
experience in the ER…

Angels in the ER

Miracles in the ER

Angels on the Night Shift

Angels on Call

Angels and Heroes

Notes from a Doctor's Pocket

To learn more about Harvest House books and
to read sample chapters, visit our website:

www.harvesthousepublishers.com

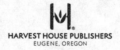

HARVEST HOUSE PUBLISHERS
EUGENE, OREGON